"THIS IS ONE OF THE MOST IMPORTANT AND BEAUTIFUL
BOOKS I HAVE EVER READ. . . . THE BOOK IS WRITTEN
WITH THE PASSION OF A MAN WHO NOT ONLY CARES
BUT KNOWS."
—Colin Turnbull

"Pearce may just blow a big enough hole in our ideas about
childhood to let some more innocence and 'fantasy' back into
our lives. A strong, reasoned book that details the wisdom of
childhood and shows why and how we must learn from children."

—Sam Keen, author of
Fire in the Belly

"A RICH BOOK . . . I hope it will help people to open the
aperture of their logical, rational minds."
—Frederick Leboyer

"YOU CAN'T HELP BUT BE INSPIRED."
—*Minneapolis Star-Tribune*

JOSEPH CHILTON PEARCE is the father of five children and
the author of *The Crack in the Cosmic Egg, Exploring the Crack
in the Cosmic Egg, The Bond of Power,* and *The Magical Child
Matures.* A former humanities teacher, he now devotes his time
to lecturing and writing.

Magical Child

JOSEPH CHILTON PEARCE

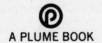

A PLUME BOOK

Dedicated to Karen

PLUME
Published by the Penguin Group
Penguin Books USA Inc., 375 Hudson Street, New York, New York 10014, U.S.A.
Penguin Books Ltd, 27 Wrights Lane, London W8 5TZ, England
Penguin Books Australia Ltd, Ringwood, Victoria, Australia
Penguin Books Canada Ltd, 10 Alcorn Avenue, Toronto, Ontario, Canada M4V 3B2
Penguin Books (N.Z.) Ltd, 182-190 Wairau Road, Auckland 10, New Zealand

Penguin Books Ltd, Registered Offices: Harmondsworth, Middlesex, England

Published by Plume, an imprint of Dutton Signet, a division of Penguin Books USA Inc.
Previously published in a Dutton edition.

First Plume Printing, March, 1992
20 19 18 17 16 15

Copyright © Joseph Chilton Pearce, 1977

 REGISTERED TRADEMARK—MARCA REGISTRADA

LIBRARY OF CONGRESS CATALOGING-IN-PUBLICATION DATA
Pearce, Joseph Chilton.
    Magical child / Joseph Chilton Pearce.
        p.   cm.
    Includes bibliographical references and index.
    ISBN 0-452-26789-7
    1. Child psychology. 2. Child rearing. I. Title.
BF721.P362   1992
155.4'13—dc20   91-36485
                                                     CIP

Printed in the United States of America

BOOKS ARE AVAILABLE AT QUANTITY DISCOUNTS WHEN USED TO PROMOTE PRODUCTS OR SERVICES.
FOR INFORMATION PLEASE WRITE TO PREMIUM MARKETING DIVISION, PENGUIN BOOKS USA INC.,
375 HUDSON STREET, NEW YORK, NEW YORK 10014.

Contents

Contents

Acknowledgments

Many people contributed to this work, sending me the majority of the books, research papers, and articles I have used. My sincere thanks to all of them. Thanks to Ralph and Judy Blum, who introduced E. P. Dutton's senior editor Bill Whitehead to a sketch of the original material. Sincerest thanks to Bill and to Pat Murray, whose insight penetrated my turgid prose, glimpsed the magical child there, and patiently worked to clarify that glimpse. My thanks to Nancie Brown, who managed the seminars through which the material achieved its synthesis. Thanks to George and Ruth Barati for my residency at the Montalvo Center for the Arts in Saratoga, California, the shelter under which much of this was written. Thanks to Katherine Barkeley, who tempered my extreme judgments and gave insight into motherhood at its finest. Finally, my dedication to Karen Hinds speaks of more than thanks.

Preface

The material in this book has led me to a position so at odds with current opinion about the child mind and human intelligence that I have been at some loss to bridge the gap. At issue is a biological plan for the growth of intelligence, a genetic encoding within us that we ignore, damage, and even destroy. The mind-brain is designed for astonishing capacities, but its development is based on the infant and child constructing a knowledge of the world as it actually is. Children are unable to construct this foundation because we unknowingly inflict on them an anxiety-conditioned view of the world (as it was unknowingly inflicted on us). Childhood is a battleground between the biological plan's *intent*, which drives the child from within, and our anxious *intentions*, pressing the child from without.

Nature has provided that the human child be more dependent on a caretaker, for a longer period of time, than any other species. If parents and society honored nature's purpose behind this long dependency and slow maturation, the child would discover and respond to the world without concern for the utility or value of his/her discovery. If the child were allowed to develop this natural world view, logical maturation would develop a utility, value, and ability almost beyond our imagination. Children throughout other parts of the world do, in fact, continually display abilities far beyond our accepted norms, though not for long.

I thought at first to write a simple outline of the biological plan as my understanding of it has unfolded over these years. But the material would not let me rest with that. Critical issues tumbled in: What is going so wrong in all technological countries today that infantile autism and brain damage are increasing at an epidemic rate, that childhood suicides are increasing yearly, that growing numbers of parents are beating infants and tiny children to death, that schooling is becoming increasingly unproductive, traumatic, even hazardous and improbable to maintain, and so on? I found that none of these problems, isolated to itself, is solvable. And I found that we make a serious error if we think children are only reflecting the tensions of the adult world. Rather, it may be the reverse. The issue is the nature of the child mind, human intelligence, and our biological connections with the earth system on which the development of the mind-brain depends. Until this issue is clarified and corrected, our problems can only multiply.

After working on this manuscript for a year or so, I felt it would be productive to lecture on the subject, to get feedback from parents, teachers, professionals, or whoever might be interested. The lectures grew to three-day seminars and proved of great value as a source of constant correctives, balancing theory and everyday reality and providing dozens of research sources that I might otherwise never have found. Above all, these lectures and seminars have given me a near shock wave of profound affirmative response, from many different parts of the country, to the ideas set forth in this book.

As the father of five children; as an adult who has a clear recollection of the impressions, states of mind, and expectancies of my own early years; and as a teacher in both college and public school, I had some tangible background to relate to the often abstract studies of the child, the mind-brain, and reality. I was not prepared, though, for what formed as the material broke through to me with connections and meanings I had only dimly suspected. At one point, I felt that the book was impossible for me to do, that the implications were too vast and too sad to articulate.—I underwent some depression when I began to see the potential of the child and the monumental tragedy that befalls us anew with each generation. I knew guilt over my own experience as a father and nostalgia over the loss of potential I had once felt so keenly. Only by delving as completely into the material as was possible for me did I finally see why I was *not* guilty, why none of us is or was, and why blame is largely fruitless. Once I had achieved this insight, the material showed me the extraordinary and profound potential and hope that an understanding of the child's (and our own) mind-brain holds.

Because I am writing this book as a parent to parents, a teacher to teachers, and a human concerned about the reintegration of self and child, I will avoid, as far as possible, technical terms or explanations. My sole concern is to outline the biological plan and how it is damaged, and I use any material that is helpful. The work of Jean Piaget, for instance, is one of my foundation blocks, yet I have used his theory and materials selectively as it aided my purpose. It will take us generations to appreciate the enormous scope of the work of this Swiss biologist turned psychologist. He spent some forty-five years observing the growth of intelligence in hundreds of children, and I find his work an invaluable source, guide, and model. It was, in fact, Piaget's concern over so-called magical thinking in children that proved a valuable clue and eventually gave me the title of this work. Yet, I often use his material in ways almost opposite to his own viewpoints. For the sake of brevity, I do so without explanation, argument, or apology (other than right here).

As a biologist, Piaget felt that psychology had erred by starting with the grown human and working backward to the child, carrying into research the biases and viewpoints of a mature logic. The end product of a biological organism, he said, is not the best place to start if you want to understand that organism. You must start your research at the beginning of that life and let the creature show you as it grows. Piaget found that the child had to build his or her own intellectual knowledge for interpreting and physically responding to the world. He found the infant driven from within, with a nonvolitional intent, to make the necessary physical interactions with the world. Piaget called the results the child's *structure of knowledge.* We sometimes refer to this as our *world view,* that is, the way the brain organizes its incoming information and makes an intelligent response.

Piaget found that the child goes through clear developmental stages in this growth of intelligence, stages that parallel physical growth. He found that the child's brain system and structure of knowledge undergo specific transitions on a kind of timed maturational basis. At each of these shifts, the brain then processes its information in new ways and develops new ways for interacting with a larger experience. These shifts of logic, according to Piaget, are genetically determined and occur in all children in the same sequence at about the same age—much as physical growth does, I might add.

Many people have argued against this position, particularly in this country. Jerome Bruner feels that any subject can be taught at almost any time if it is cast in a proper framework and that the stage-specific nature of learning Piaget outlines is artificially binding. Most educators have followed

Bruner and his call for earlier and earlier academic experience and training.
The People's Republic of China has been scornful of Piaget, insisting that
their children are learning abstract academic subjects very early. (But the
long-range results of China's recent experiments remain to be seen.) In the
following pages, I will concern myself with these theories counter to Piaget
only as I see them acting against the unfolding of the biological plan, not
as they relate to Piaget, whose work will stand on its own merit.

Recently, Herman Epstein, the Brandeis University biophysicist, has
found evidence of periodic brain-growth spurts in all children at about the
same stages in their development. At these periods, the brain actually grows
new biological materials for learning. These spurts occur roughly every four
years, all but one coinciding with Piaget's periods of logical transition.
Brain-growth spurts seem genetically predetermined in the same way that
Piaget's developmental stages do, and I take it as obvious that these are all
part of an integral genetic coding for the growth of intelligence.

The theory of development presented by Piaget and Epstein offers a
model in which nearly all the problems of childhood and eventual adulthood can take on new meaning. But this is the case only if we take into
consideration, and go around, Piaget's own bias, a point of view that was
almost inevitable for a twentieth-century scientist. The prejudice distinctly
qualifying his observations was his attitude toward the characteristic he
calls *magical thinking*. In this he shared the conventional view of other
researchers who refer to the child's *wish thinking, fantasizing,* or *autistic
thinking* (in the original meaning of that term) as a self-enclosed thought
that doesn't bother to check against reality. In brief, magical thinking
implies that some connection exists between thought and reality, that thinking enters into and can influence the actual world. Child thought is based
on this attitude for the first seven or eight years. The central question of
psychologies and educational research has been: How can the child be made
to attend to reality? Or how can we make the child abandon magical
thinking?

Each generation uses its children to its own ends, Otto Rank once
claimed, and magical thinking has been one of the stumbling blocks to using
our children as we would like to in service to our technology. Has nature,
then, made a monumental error in creating a child who compulsively
spends most of his or her time in the apparently nonproductive and even
antisurvival activities of fantasy, magical thinking, and play? The implicit,
almost axiomatic answer of our whole modern treatment of children has
been: *Yes,* nature has apparently so erred, in spite of the fact that this seems
to go against the entire thrust and fabric of evolutionary adaptation and

selection. But the child's world has recently been collapsing almost as fast as our adult one. Is it not possible that our ideas of the child and nature are in error instead?

Piaget's primary interest and unconscious bias were in the development of rational scientific thought, the kind of thinking that makes great university material. His brilliant observational analysis of the development of such thinking is of immense worth, but something profoundly significant is missing. Recently, split-brain research has led to a theory of a dual functioning of the brain according to left and right hemispheres. Some researchers have decided that Piaget's type of thinking (and therefore his results) stems from *left-brain thinking*, the ordinary, linear, rational, digital thinking so typical of this century. So a counterswing is now under way to promote the education of the other half of the brain. Our ills, say the leaders of this trend, are due to overeducating the left brain. Thus, schools should incorporate right-brain curricula. I cringe at the thought.

The clue lies with the child's universal compulsion to play and fantasize. Researchers state that the infant makes no random or useless movements; from the beginning every action has meaning, purpose, and design. In the same way, if all children compulsively spend the bulk of their time in some activity, then that activity must play a major role in genetic organization. Fantasy play and magical thinking cannot be errors of nature or examples of a faulty child logic needing adult correction because no species could survive with such a built-in contradiction.

What I have done is to take the liberty of using Piaget's research and terms as a basis for examining the child's experience. But I have included those magical areas found unacceptable to academic thought. Once all aspects of the child's experience are examined as natural and meaningful, Piaget's own developmental theory takes on dimensions far beyond, yet still encompassing, his own interests. Concern for the viewpoints of the various specialists whose domain I encroach upon is theirs, not mine. If I have glossed over some points, ignored minor discrepancies, used or misused materials selectively, so be it. My task has been to sketch the picture of the child's mind and nature's plan for intelligence. This is a large terrain, and discrepancies are probably inevitable. But I stand by my sketch of human intelligence and intend this book to be an aid in the correction of a monstrous misunderstanding.

Part I

The
Monstrous
Misunderstanding

Chapter 1

Promise Given:
Magnificent Heritage

The human mind-brain system is designed for functions radically different from and broader than its current uses. An astonishing capacity for creative power is built into our genes, ready to unfold. Our innate capacities of mind are nothing less than miraculous, and we are born with a driving intent to express this capacity.

From the beginning, nature's emphasis is on the mind-brain. When an infant is born, his/her brain is one-fourth its final, mature size, while the body is only one-twentieth its final size. The brain is the most complex organism known to exist in this universe, and although research has made impressive and gigantic strides in recent years, the mystery of the mind grows correspondingly deeper and richer.

Current opinion suggests that we use only a small portion of our brain capacity. This book explores both why we fail to utilize our brains fully and what a full utilization might mean for us. We receive continual, if sporadic, reports of brain usage and resulting phenomena that fall outside current notions of human possibility. We tend to dismiss these reports because we have no framework into which to fit them, no criteria for giving them meaning. And not incidentally, this continual stream of excluded phenomena calls our systems of belief into question.

The existence of a genetically planned development of the body's physical growth is apparent. We even know how nature programs this growth through DNA genetic coding. All infants and children of all cultures follow the same pattern of body development and at about the same rate of maturation. Baby teeth, six-year molars, twelve-year molars, genital sexuality, and so on appear at about the same time in all countries and among all races. We are not, thank God, responsible for the order or timing of this unfolding. All we are called upon to do is nurture the genetic plan, not supplant it.

This book discusses a corresponding, beautifully coordinated biological plan for the development of intelligence. Indeed, we find that body growth, so self-evident, follows the needs of the mind-brain's development in perfect synchrony. To allow full development of intelligence, we must acknowledge and cooperate with this biological plan. In so doing, we will find that most of our current problems with infants and children will never materialize. For our problems are largely man-made, caused by ignoring nature's plan. Nature herself worked out all problems aeons ago.

Just as no two sets of fingerprints are alike, the genetic plan for the development of intelligence is unique to every human. Yet, most human infants are born with essentially the same brain mechanisms. Even a large difference in brain size does not fully determine the scope of intelligence. Anatole France, with his tiny braincase, and Turgenev, with his huge one, are the classical examples. Nature may not endow some few chosen brains with superiority, as we have long thought. Back in 1938, for instance, Harold Skeels, of the University of Iowa, was nearly drummed out of the American Psychological Association for his studies suggesting that I.Q. (the intelligence quotient of a person) was directly related to environmental conditions, particularly the nurturings of home and family. For everyone knew that intelligence was innate, a fixed genetic factor. Everyone was tragically wrong, of course, and eventually Skeels was recognized. Intelligence, like the body, can be injured or nurtured, stimulated or starved.

Barriers to intelligence have long since been winnowed out by nature because nature does not program for failure. Nature programs for success and has thus built a vast and awesome program for success into our genes. Nature also programs the parent to respond with the precise nurturings needed. What she cannot program is parental failure to nurture the infant-child.

Nature programs every new brain system for maximum potential. To say that every child is a potential genius may sound ridiculous and even cruel, but to take current statistical norms as the standard or natural for the child is far more ridiculous and surely more cruel.

Our ancestors have been on this earth for several million years, and even at our appearance here, life had been producing thinking organisms for 3 billion years. Ours is an astonishing heritage; we contain within our small skulls the culmination of these aeons of slow and steady brain evolution. To understand the nature of the mind-brain, we must first grasp the awesome stretch of time our living earth has spent in genetic-code experimentation leading to our present state.

In her 3-billion-year preparation for us, life moved from simple thinking forms to ever more complex ones. This movement still takes place through a slow evolution, working through selection and through quantum jumps of possibility. And in the marvelous economy of nature, nothing is lost. Each progression life makes toward greater intelligence encompasses all previous gains. Our skulls, for instance, contain an old brain and a new brain. Our old brains are made of what is called the *reptilian brain* that is some 200 to 300 million years old (i.e., it was developed and perfected that long ago), and an *old mammalian brain* that is nearly as ancient. And it is through this system that we inherit the gains of the past.

We have, as well, the new brain, or *neocortex*. Nature experimented with the size of this new brain time and again before settling on our particular dimensions. We have a far greater amount of this gray matter than lower animals, yet nowhere near so much as the giant whales and some dolphins. The amount we have is just what we need for certain goals nature has in mind, such as our dominion over the earth.

Furthermore, intelligence is not assigned only to the brain and nervous system. Every cell of our bodies is an intelligence of staggering complexity, and every cell acts intelligently.[1] The mind-brain-body is a wonderful array of intelligences ranging from the simpler life forms of the cell and old brain to the most complex (neocortex). Each human being contains the patterns of all thinking forms developed over the millennia.

There are no limits to the possibilities within genetic coding.[2] Nature can program an indefinite amount of information and ability into a brain system, even quite simple and tiny ones. Consider the homing pigeon, which can find its way back over hundreds of miles. Its tiny brain appears to have a knowledge of the magnetic lines of force surrounding the earth, and it navigates by means of this built-in knowledge. Eels and salmon can find their way unerringly through thousands of miles of ocean, up hundreds of miles of fresh water, to the very brook from which they came as fingerlings. They appear to have a built-in map of the world and an equal ability to chart their course accurately. Most animal species seem to have complex preprogrammed information about the world and about how to move successfully in it. All they need at birth is exposure to that world for these innate programs to be quickly activated and brought into play. The result is a rapid autonomy; they mature and can take care of themselves in a short time.

Brain researchers are now beginning to consider the brain as a form of *hologram.* A hologram is a kind of photography that contains the entire photograph within any part or piece of the whole. (You must see this to believe it.) There are many uncanny properties of holography, but this phenomenon of the whole within the part is the property that seems similar to the brain. For example, take a hologram plate of a vase of flowers, and break that plate in half. You do not have a picture of two halves of a vase; each half is still the complete picture. Break the plate into quarters, and you will have four complete pictures, and so on, down to small fragments. The problem is that the picture gets fuzzier at each reduction. A tiny piece still contains the whole picture, but the clarity is gone.

When we speak of the brain as a hologram, we mean that any part of the brain, even a single thinking cell, reflects or encompasses the workings of the total brain. An even more intriguing implication is that the brain may be a hologram of the entire planet earth. That is, just as you can divide a holographic plate and find the whole picture in any piece, so the brain can be considered just such a piece of the earth, reflecting within it the picture or workings of the whole life system. The human brain may be a kind of microminiature replica of the living planet itself, just rather fuzzy at the edges, needing clarification.

The model of the brain as hologram automatically implies a further extension of the hologram notion. The brain may be a hologram of the planet earth, but that planet itself must then be a hologram. (Indeed, just this model has been suggested by some of our greatest brain researchers.[3]) So to use this model, we can consider our brains pieces of the earth hologram, just as any and all parts of the earth are pieces of a greater hologram. This is something that mystics and poets have alluded to down through the ages, as when William Blake wrote, "To see the world in a grain of sand. . . ."

At birth, the brain, as a hologram fragment, must have exposure to and interact with the earth hologram to achieve clarity, to bring the brain's picture into focus, so to speak. Confine a newly born brain and prevent interaction with the earth, and no clarification can take place. That creature will be retarded and helpless. If a kitten spends his first few critical weeks of development in a compartment with vertically striped walls, the grown cat will be able to see only those objects of a vertical nature.[4] He will avoid the legs of a chair perfectly well but will run smack into the horizontal rungs.

The speed and efficiency with which the newborn brain hologram achieves its clarity by interaction with the earth hologram depends upon how extensive a reflection of the total earth hologram that brain contains. Those brains reflecting highly specific aspects of the earth, such as the brain of a homing pigeon or a bee, achieve rapid autonomy. The greater the potential content of the brain hologram, the slower the process of clarification. The brain achieves its clarity of operations only through interacting with or moving into physical touch with the living earth itself, which is to say that the hologram fragment achieves its clarity by interacting with the total hologram. To the extent the newborn is allowed interaction with the earth, to that extent the brain clarifies its own portion of the picture.

Life has moved from simple to ever more complex thinking forms. To use our hologram model (as I shall throughout), I would say that life has moved from highly specific and limited (thus simpler) holograms to ever more complete and complex ones. Nature *could* program an infinite amount of information and ability into a brain system, but she is selective in the particular nature of any hologram brain. The homing pigeon has marvelous capacities, but it is only a narrow fragment of the total earth picture. Eels and salmon have a marvelous navigation but are, after all, not very adaptable or flexible. We can easily figure out their particular preprogramming, predict the journey built into their world map, set up nets, and wipe them out. Nature programs according to an intricate ecological balance. Each bit of the hologram system interacts with the total for precise functions; every creature fits into the balance with meaning, purpose, and design.

Life appears to keep many of her experimental creatures if they fit this balance successfully; others she discards as she moves on toward certain goals. In moving from simpler to more complex forms, life created an interacting system of stability yet continued moving toward more advanced brains, or more complete holograms of her total experience. Of course, her total always includes the interacting balance of all the life forms. She builds in a capacity for the clarifying of her ever more extensive and complete holograms through an ever more extensive capacity for physical interaction with the total.

In moving from simpler to more complex thinkings organs, life's growth has been toward a more open intelligence and a more flexible logic. The more open the intelligence, the greater the totality of the earth that hologram can express. Furthermore, an open intelligence is one that can structure a knowledge of an increasing amount of experience and compute the widening range of information gained by that experience. By flexible logic, I mean a brain system that can differentiate between its experiences, combine them, and synthesize new ways to interact with more complex kinds of experience. Open intelligence and flexible logic combine so that the more we learn through personal experience, the more we *can* learn; the more phenomena and events with which we interact, the greater our ability for more complex interactions. And the design of nature in the combination of an open intelligence and flexible logic is to get beyond the specific limitations of the earth hologram itself; that is, in the human system, life has evolved a way for getting beyond the restrictions of holograms in general. What this means is the subject of this book. Each animal species is able to interact with the earth within certain strict limits. Lower brains are not holograms of the whole earth, only of certain aspects of that earth. The simpler the brain, the more specific its programming and the more readily it can efficiently interact with the earth. The newborn baby chick can immediately recognize and peck at seeds of the proper shape and size. The frog sees only those movements in his environment that relate to his food supply and/or safety. The larger and more elaborate the brain, the wider the hologram effect of that species and the greater its intelligence or ability to interact.

As we move up the evolutionary scale, we find not only larger old brains, carrying larger portions of the earth hologram, but also the so-called silent areas of the brain, a new kind of brain matter that does not seem to be a preprogrammed part of the hologram. This new brain material, the neocortex, is the computer part of the brain. It appears to be able to solve problems that cannot be programmed as fixed information. This is the part of the brain that develops logic. The higher apes have more of this new-brain material than lower animals and prove able to learn more and even interact creatively. (Recently, several chimpanzees have been taught to read and make sentences.) Even so, much of their brain is programmed for specific interactions with the earth and needs only a brief exposure to that earth for the programs to be fully activated. This gives quick autonomy but limited capacities.

Human infants have a long, slow development of autonomy. They are more helpless for a longer period of time than infants of any other species. There are two reasons for this (that I know of), and these will prove decisive in responding to the child appropriately: First, within the older-brain systems, we almost surely carry the information and ability acquired through all the earth's history. This preprogramming encompasses the total life hologram and its knowledge. The vastness of this programming means that none of its information is specific. Human infants are not limited to certain parts of the earth to activate their programming. The Eskimo, in his environment of ice and snow, can achieve as full an intellectual development as the Balinese or Australian can in their strikingly different worlds. Lack of specificity means that autonomy, that combination of knowledge and ability, takes quite a long time to develop.[5]

Second, there is a striking difference between the older, genetically programmed brain systems and the new, unprogrammed brain. And in this difference lies the resolution of the long argument concerning "nature versus nurture," which is an argument about whether we have information built in or whether we must acquire all our information. (One school of thought argues that the prolonged helplessness of the infant-child permits the child to be taught our cumulative social knowledge, lest he remain animallike. This position is no longer tenable.)

The reason for the long period of dependency is that the infant-child must structure his/her own knowledge of the world, and s/he must do this almost from scratch. Paradoxically, the infant is born into this world with a brain system that may be a hologram of the entire earth system. The paradox is resolved when we consider that it is the old-brain system, with its reptilian and old-mammalian brains, that represents the life hologram. The new brain, the infant's future computer, is the blank slate.

Were we to operate entirely out of the old-brain system (as indeed we do at first), we would be as purely instinctive as the lower species. We would have neither an open intelligence nor a flexible logic; we would have no creativity or individual personality. Our old-brain hologram is of such vast dimensions that its outlines are fuzzy, undifferentiated, and nonspecific. Any specifics from this total must be slowly brought into play through physical interaction. The whole riddle of development and the vast difference between man and animal center on the method of articulation or clarification of the potential carried in the old-brain system.

What happens, in brief, is that the old brain's hologram content is only *in potentia* and must be structured as actual workable knowledge in the new-brain system, which will become the decision-making, computer area. In the old brain, such knowledge would lead only to a reflexive, instinctual pattern of action. But when it is translated as structured knowledge in the new brain, we develop conscious and flexible action, with eventual creativity.

The transfer from old-brain potential to new-brain actuality takes place through the infant-child's muscular body movements. The older-brain systems run the physical body, dictating or activating the actual body movements of the child. The opening stages of the biological plan rest entirely on a preprogrammed plan for moving that infant-child's body in a prescribed manner. These early body movements impell (literally drive or propel) the child into physical interactions with whatever material substance of this earth is available to him/her and equally into the physical principles, the laws of cause and effect, by which this earth operates.

These physical interactions with the world bring about a simultaneous patterning of that particular experience in the infant-child's new-brain system. Thus, the child's knowledge structure builds out of almost infinitely varied possibilities, yet proves to be a knowledge of the living earth as it actually operates. Then, through a marvelous function of logical feedback, that computer-brain system develops volitional control over the knowledge structured, develops the ability to decide freely between alternatives for interaction, develops the ability to interact creatively with the world through the structure of knowledge built up about that world, and eventually can even transform parts of that world itself, as needed for security and well-being.

Jerome Bruner observed that the infant-child's "intent precedes the ability to do." Every infant and child shows an intent to perform some act, such as talking or walking or sitting up, long before s/he can actually do so. The infant in the crib makes clumsy, jerking thrusts toward an object long before s/he succeeds in correctly aiming toward and grasping that object; s/he makes preliminary gestures toward turning over long before s/he succeeds; s/he starts trying to sit up before s/he can.

It is easy enough to observe this intent, so crude in its initial movements, but where does it come from? It does not come from imitation. The infant-child might observe the parent sitting up, walking, and so on, but the child does not observe all the preliminary movements that s/he must go through to accomplish that act. Furthermore, the blind child, for whom visual imitation is not possible, will show the same rough gestures of intent. What propels that infant body to make those movements? Instincts, we say. But what is an instinct? An instinct is some nonvolitional reflexive action that operates largely autonomously, that is, without volitional prompting. Sucking on a nipple is such a built-in action. Now surely *intent* operates as an instinct, and surely it arises from the old-brain system, possibly from the cerebellum (a large organ that seems to be involved in body movement). But intent differs from instinct in that it is translated into volitional, conscious activity generated from the computer areas of the brain.

We adults move through our own volition. We decide to move, walk, or whatever, and our body-knowing just does it for us. Such volitional action almost surely comes from new-brain decisions or acts in conjunction with older-brain functions controlling the body. But this is not the case with the infant or child. S/he has no volition. The infant-child has only *intent,* and this intent comes from older-brain processes. The surprising and disturbing fact about the early child is that for the first three years or so, s/he has no volitional control, no will, in the adult sense. That child is moved by his/her intent much as a puppet is moved by its strings. Intent, arising from programmed, autonomic old-brain controls, literally impels that body into interaction with the physical world. The early child cannot knowingly disobey a parent or willfully misbehave. The early child can only obey the inborn intent that moves him/her.

The intent to do has little or no content; that is, intent contains nothing specific, no actual concrete knowledge. The intent is simply an impulse that moves the child's body in its initial crude attempts to interact with the actual world. These body movements and the sensory experiences accompanying or resulting from them are recorded, for lack of a better term, in the form of patterns or tracings of action within the rhythmic patterns in the new brain's thinking cells. To put it crudely, when the nursing infant reaches up and touches the mother's face, the resulting sensory information etches into the new brain in coordination with the particular body movements giving that kind of information. The attempt to sit up makes an attempted pattern in the new brain. Through his/her repeated efforts, the infant's intent etches in these brain patterns more securely; the rhythmic patterning carrying that kind of information and coordination gets smoother, and the body's responses grow correspondingly smoother and surer. And when sitting up is complete or successful, the pattern is complete and successful.

The intent that drives the child for the first few years is that of physical interaction with all the possible contents of the living earth (its creatures, phenomena, experiences, and things) and, above all, its principles and laws of interaction. These principles are quite practical and mundane, such as "fall down, go boom," and "fire means burn." Each physical contact the child makes brings about a corresponding patterning, or learning, in his/her new brain. These patterns and the relationships between them that are made through regulatory feedback then grow as the child's *structure of knowledge,* or world view. The story of development for the first four or five years is the structuring of these brain patterns from sensory experience and the resulting feedback and synthesis that take place within the brain.

Development is the interaction of the intent within and the content without. Intent moves the child toward interaction with content out there. The intent within must always be given its content from without. The more extensive and complete the child's interaction with the content of the world out there, the more extensive the resulting structure of knowledge within.

The greater that structure, the greater the possibilities for internal feedback, synthesis, and volitional control and so the greater the child's ability to interact with more content from without. Through logical feedback, the child eventually develops a volitional control over his/her own activities and later on in life even volitional control over his/her own brain activities.

Intelligence is the ability to interact, and this ability can grow only by interacting with new phenomena, that is, by moving from that which is known into that which is not known. Although this seems obvious, this movement from the known to the unknown proves to be both the key and the stumbling block to development. Most intellectual crippling comes from the failure to observe the balance of this movement. In our anxieties, we fail to allow the child a continual interaction with the phenomena of this earth on a full-dimensional level (which means with all five of his/her body senses); and at the same time, we rush the child into contact with phenomena not appropriate to his/her stage of biological development. That is, either we block the child's movement into the unknown and so block intellectual growth, or we propel the child into inappropriate experience.

From birth, the growth of intelligence is a progression from the concrete toward the abstract. By concrete, I mean the physical substance of this living earth (its rocks, trees, people, winds, things) and its principles (such as "fall down, go boom" and "fire means burn"). By abstract, I mean the products of the mind-brain's own creativity (thoughts and ideas) rather than the actual material substance of the earth. Just as evolution has been a movement toward more complex thinking forms, the growth of thinking is a movement from concrete thought (knowledge of, and ability to respond to, the physical events of the earth) toward purely abstract phenomena (the thoughts occurring within the mind-brain itself).

All thinking arises out of concreteness, which means out of the brain patterns resulting from actual body movements of interacting with actual things. But thinking then moves toward autonomy, that is, moves toward independence of those concrete patterns or physical principles. This progression toward pure thought is itself genetically programmed and unfolds in neat, sequential stages. To nurture intelligence in the young is to honor this progression from concreteness toward abstraction. This means that intelligence must first be educated in an accurate and full interaction with the earth as it is in order that the mind-brain might structure a knowledge of this earth. This *is* physical knowledge, or basic body-knowing. Only out of this kind of knowing can abstract thought develop, such as an understanding of the law of gravity rather than "fall down, go boom" or the laws of thermodynamics rather than "hot, don't touch."

Flexible logic depends on the ability to differentiate between experiences and then group them into useful categories. This differentiation begins quite early in life and is the function of *regulatory feedback*. One automatic and natural result of this differentiation is the development of a conscious, personal awareness, a sense of individuality. This leads to a concern for physical welfare that is qualitatively different from that of the more un-differentiated mind-brains of lower species. Therefore, a method or proce-dure for protection of our physical body must automatically be a part of the development of intelligence if the mind is eventually to move beyond concrete concerns, that is, to move from concreteness toward abstraction, concrete concerns such as physical safety must be accomplished and gotten behind one.

The same qualification holds for the development of personality itself, which is also an automatic result of the logic of differentiation. We hear that the human is the only creature who seems to know s/he must die. The same logic of differentiation that gives us our individual consciousness leads us to our awareness of personal death. If not met with appropriate content and abilities, this awareness would lead to an anxiety blocking further move-ment into pure abstraction. But life would not have spent such an astonish-ingly long period of time developing a logic that, in turn, develops individu-ality and awareness of death as personal only to mock the resulting individual with his/her own mortality. Rather, the movement for a logic of survival through adaptability has led to the creation of *both* individual consciousness and the means for a survival of that consciousness. Anything less would be a contradiction of terms within the evolution of intelligence.

There are three levels of adaptability and survival, and the means for these unfold sequentially in the biological plan: Physical survival unfolds through creative interactions with the world; species survival unfolds through genital sexuality; and personal survival unfolds through the devel-opment of pure abstract thought.

For quite a while now, academic thought has insisted that nature bred our hairless, vulnerable bodies (perhaps accidentally) and that that vulnera-bility forced *us* to evolve our great brain system in order to make tools to protect our vulnerable bodies. This belief is so ingrained that we actually believe that only through tools (houses, clothes, weapons, machinery, writ-ing, books) can we survive. We assume that tool usage is the real mark of intelligence and set up tool capacity (including writing as a tool) as the final criteria for intelligence. We mold young minds accordingly, centering the training of children on tool usage and the complex abstract systems we have evolved out of such usage. Finally, we conclude that without this engineered tinkering with the mind of the early child, that child would be as a beast of the field, without language, thought, writing, or—horrors—tools.

The extent of this error will occupy this book, but in no way am I going to attack technological achievments. In no way would I call (even if I could) for a return to the forests primeval. The human was not meant to live in the wilderness. On the other hand, the current breakdown of social life clearly shows that we were not meant to live in the strange nightmare world of a city. Humans are designed to live in the garden. To live in the garden, we must tend that garden. We must be good stewards of our resources and exercise careful dominion over them. Tools could be an adjunct to this stewardship over the earth. We get in serious difficulties when we substitute mechanics for personal power, for they are qualitatively different functions.

Nikos Tinbergen devoted two-thirds of his 1973 Nobel laureate speech to the epidemic increase in infantile autism, an epidemic breaking out in all the technological countries of the world. Autism is the cruelest and most nearly hopeless of all childhood psychoses (although it is hardly even in the simple category of a psychosis). Childhood schizophrenia is also on the rise, as are silent crib deaths, brain damage, hyperactivity dysfunction, mental retardation, and learning disabilities. Nor are we just making better diagnoses; the number of damaged children is rapidly increasing all about us. Achievement scoring in the American schools has been on a sharp decline for a decade. Within the short period from 1974 to 1976, structure and discipline within the schools have suffered a sharp, decided decline. Teachers of a long and successful standing are folding up physically and mentally, unable to cope with the random meaninglessness. Suicides committed by children under fourteen years of age have increased many hundreds of times in the past fifteen years. And now we have a new and strange breakdown of the body's metabolism called *anorexia nervosa,* which strikes down teenagers, particularly girls.

Our children have been signaling us for years that things are critically wrong for them. In our anxiety-ridden concern to "equip them fully for life," we have been deaf and blind to their distress calls. And now our training techniques, our teaching systems, our behavior modifications and motivations are turning into chaos, both for our children and for ourselves. Perhaps at this critical point for the survival of the species, we can do more than make another futile gesture toward patching up the holes in our exhausted system of ideas. Perhaps we can seize this cubic centimeter of chance that history is giving us and move, not just to correct some of the more blatant and tragic errors we have made with children, not just to curb the battered-child syndrome, but actually to turn again to that 3-billion-year development lying within us, that uncanny wisdom of the body clearly programmed into the child as unbending intent. In learning to learn again, we can learn of this wisdom and allow our children (and so ourselves) to become the free, whole individuals this good earth has prepared us to be.

Chapter 2

Matrix Shifts:
Known to Unknown

Matrix is the Latin word for womb. From that word, we get the words *matter, material, mater, mother,* and so on. These refer to the basic stuff, the physical substance, out of which life is derived.

The womb offers three things to a newly forming life: a source of possibility, a source of energy to explore that possibility, and a safe place within which that exploration can take place. Whenever these three needs are met, we have a matrix. And the growth of intelligence takes place by utilizing the energy given to explore the possibilities given while standing in the safe space given by the matrix.

A matrix is always essentially female by nature. The male sperm must quickly find refuge in the female egg or perish. The egg matrix is given the energy, possibility, and safe space of the womb matrix within the mother matrix (who stands within the earth matrix). After an infant is born from the womb, the mother becomes the source of energy, the possibility, and the safe place on which to stand, so mother rightly means matrix. Later in development, the earth itself should become the matrix, and we have always referred to mother earth. Nature was always considered the general spirit of the earth's life and was called mother nature or matrix.

The biological plan for the development of intelligence is based on a series of matrix formations and shifts; that is, human beings are designed to grow in intelligence by learning about, and gaining ability to interact with, one source of energy, possibility, and security after another. The sequence is from early concrete matrices to ever more abstract ones, that is, from the matrix of our given life substance to the matrix of pure creative thought. Each matrix shift propels us into another set of unknown, unpredictable experiences, which is the way intelligence grows. Each matrix shift is both a kind of birth because we move into greater possibilities and a kind of death because the old matrix must be given up in order to move into the new.

These matrix shifts follow a set cycle. First, the mind-brain must structure its knowledge of its matrix. This structuring has its own *cycle of competence* (or pattern of growth), which I will discuss in Chapter 9, and is accomplished through sensory interaction with the actual content and possibilities of that matrix. The matrix always furnishes the energy necessary for this exploration, and the matrix is, of course, the safe place or protective environment in which the exploration can take place. For instance, the infant in utero structures a knowledge of the womb world even as the body and brain are structured. Physical and intellectual growth are designed as a perfect synchrony.

Second, the mind-brain develops bonds (forms of communication and rapport) with both its present matrix and the new matrix into which the child must eventually shift as genetic maturation unfolds. While in utero, the infant prepares for his/her eventual separation from the womb by establishing bonds of communication with the mother. (These bonds are probably partly hormonal, as well as psychobiological and below ordinary consciousness.) This bonding process provides a bridge between matrices so that the unknown of the new matrix will have sufficient points of similarity with the known of the old matrix. Then, the mind-brain can accommodate, or learn about and adapt to, the new. Nature would never (of her own choice) propel the child into a new matrix without sufficient preparation, because s/he would be unable to adapt or survive in the new. And remember that nature programs entirely for success.

Third, when we have structured a knowledge of the matrix, can move successfully within it, and have established bondings with the new matrix, we shift functionally from dependence on the known matrix and move into the next stage of development, the next matrix. We move into the new matrix only by standing on the old matrix, so to speak. For instance, the early child can move into an exploration of the world only by standing on the safe place provided by the mother. Later, after age seven, the child can move into the matrix of his/her own personal power only by standing on the safe place of the earth itself.

Fourth, having shifted matrices, we then have the possibility of a wider, more creative relationship with the former matrix. We find (*only* after leaving a matrix) that we do not lose that matrix but are able to interact with it in far more flexible and creative ways. So long as the infant is in utero, s/he is only a symbiotic extension of the mother. A flexible, creative relationship is not possible, only a relationship of total dependence. To relate creatively and so explore all possibilities, independence from the matrix must be achieved. To relate fully with the mother, the infant must leave the womb and, eventually, the dependency relation with the mother. After age seven, to relate fully with the world, the child must functionally separate from that world. (By "functionally separate," I mean within the brain's processing of information.) Each matrix is encompassed within the next matrix and thereby takes on greater possibilities.

Biologically, we are supported at each matrix shift with enhanced physical ability, a spurt of new brain growth that prepares us for new learning, and specific shifts of the brain's ways of processing information. Furthermore, intent always precedes the ability to do; that is, during any particular stage of development, nature is preparing us for the next stage. Yet, the beauty of the system is that we are conscious of none of this. All we must do is fully accept and exist within our developmental stage and respond fully to its content. This means that every stage of development is complete and perfect within itself. The three-year-old is not an incomplete five-year-old; the child is not an incomplete adult. Never are we simply on our way; always, we have arrived.

Paradoxically, of course, the child certainly *is* an incomplete adult, and we exist in a flow in which nothing can remain stationary. Everything is only preparatory to something else that is in formation, as day must fade to night and night to day. But all this is part of an infinitely contingent natural system that simply lies beyond our conscious grasp and is, in effect, none of our business. The intricacies of the 3-billion-year system are not necessarily available to, or needed by, our short-term understanding.

The progression of matrix shifts is from concreteness toward abstraction, or from the purely physical world of the womb, mother, earth, and body to the purely mental world of thought itself. The cycle unfolds according to a genetic timetable that is roughly the same in all cultures. Variations do occur in timing, but never in the sequence of progressions; that is, maturity can be somewhat speeded up (as it is among the Pygmies) or slowed down, but the stages of maturation cannot be skipped or mixed up (at least not without lots of troublemaking). Just as baby teeth come before giant twelve-year molars, so all the ramifications of concrete thought and experience must mature before abstract thought and experience can unfold. We can force certain forms of abstraction prematurely on the child in his/her concrete stage of development, but the effects are specifically damaging (even though the damage will not be detectable for several years).

The cycle of growth unfolds automatically, rather as though there are so many spins around the sun and, lo, the next set of molars appears, the next brain-growth spurt takes place, logical processing shifts, and we move into the next matrix. Apparently this time sequence is a kind of statistical probability worked out by nature over the millennia. The infant in utero requires about nine months, give or take a bit, to be ready for a matrix shift; the newborn infant requires about eight or nine months to structure a knowledge of the mother as new matrix and move out to explore the larger matrix, earth; the child requires about seven years to structure a knowledge of the earth matrix and shift from mother as safe space to earth itself; and so on.

What the biological plan does not, and apparently cannot, take into consideration is the failure of development within any particular stage. That next stage unfolds, regardless. Baby teeth arrive pretty much on schedule, as do six-year molars and so on; this physical timing is not dependent on diet (or the good graces of a dentist), although the quality or efficiency of those teeth might well be. Genital sexuality unfolds around adolescence whether or not the young person (or, God knows, the parents) is prepared for that unfolding. In the same way, matrix shifts take place automatically, whether or not a proper response and structuring has taken place to prepare for that shift.

For instance, if the mother's body is producing massive amounts of adrenal steroids during pregnancy, as a result of chronic anxiety, maltreatment, or fear, the infant in the womb automatically shares in these stress hormones; they pass right through the placenta. That infant is locked into a free-floating anxiety, a kind of permanent body stress. If you have ever undergone a fright that startles your entire body, you know the body feeling of this stress state. Consider, then, having just such a flooding of fear without any conceivable reason for it; that is what a free-floating anxiety is. Locked into this tension, the infant in utero cannot develop intellectually or establish the bonding with the mother in preparation for birth. However, nature cannot program for this variable and wait for the damaging effects of chronic stress to be removed. Growth (at least physical growth) goes right ahead while intellectual growth struggles along as best it can in its crippled state, slipping farther and farther behind. If the infant does not spontaneously abort, it will be born deficient in intelligence if not in body, highly prone to early infantile autism or childhood schizophrenia, or dys-functional in a wide variety of ways. At best, the child will have to use its intelligence to try to compensate for its deficiencies. The timed unfolding goes right ahead, and the child's deficiencies accumulate. The greater the deficiencies, the more stringently the system must compensate. Making up means remaining behind trying to get the basic pattern together. But mean-while, the wheels roll on; the intelligence meant to be fully absorbed in the present and adapting to it is back somewhere trying to get the machine working. If the first matrix formation is incomplete or insufficient, the next matrix formation will be doubly difficult. The young life is more and more jeopardized because the shifts of matrices must take place automatically. (Bear this in mind in Chapter 6, when I discuss childbirth as the most critical of all human events.)

Intelligence is the ability to interact with one's matrix. Interaction means a dynamic interchange of energy. The design of nature is that we interact with our matrix in order to interchange our energy and possibility with that of the matrix, which automatically increases and enhances our safe place on which to stand. At conception, the human organism is microscopic, but given the safe place for growth, the vast possibilities of the huge womb world, and the great energies of the mother's body to call on, that tiny organism grows at an astonishing rate. Its energy and life interchange and flow with the energy and life of its matrix and are amplified in so doing. The tiny creature gestures with its energy to its matrix, and its matrix gestures back with greatly expanded energies. The tiny body sows a wind and reaps a whirlwind, finds itself magnified thousands of times in its own energy, possibility, and security. This interaction is the growth of intelligence and body and is the pattern our entire life *should* follow. At the appointed time, when a knowledge of the matrix is completed, that new creature triggers into motion its own exodus from that matrix and moves into the infinitely larger matrix of the mother herself.

At each matrix stage, life provides that our gestures be reflected back to us by the vastly greater gestures of the matrix. The overall design is open-ended and is limited only by the individual's capacity for interaction, never by the possibilities for interaction. By its very structure, the brain's capacity for concept structuring and synthesizing can never be exhausted; and our independence and capacity of mind, designed to grow from that brain capacity, can only add to and go beyond this flexibility and freedom.

In the chapters to follow, I will trace the five matrix shifts that take place in the developmental years and some of the ways our proper maturation fails to take place. I have already offered a sketch of life in the womb as first matrix and of the shift from womb to mother at birth. Research shows that the mother is the infant-child's basis for exploration of the world itself. The reason for the child's total dependency on the parent for so long does not lie just with psychological, emotional, or sentimental causes, nor with anxiety over survival; rather, it lies with specific biological functions in the brain system. Physical interaction with the mother (or permanent caretaker) furnishes the infant with his/her basic set of brain patterns through which sensory information can be organized into perceptions. The mother *is* the infant's world, hologram, the content for his/her intent; she is the infant's power, possibility, and safe space.

The biological plan provides that the infant be given exactly the kinds of sensorimotor tools (physical capacities) needed to do one thing in the first eight to ten months of life: structure a knowledge of that mother as the matrix. Once this critical task is accomplished, nature provides that the infant be given the physical and mental tools necessary to move slowly out from that mother and explore the living world around him/her. The infant can do this fully and successfully only to the extent the mother is his/her absolutely unquestioned safe place to which s/he can always instantly return and be nurtured. Only when the infant knows that the mother matrix will not abandon him/her can that infant move into childhood with confidence and power.

The biological plan provides that the child remain squarely rooted to the mother while s/he explores and structures a knowledge of the earth matrix. This world view structuring takes some seven years to perfect. When a knowledge of the earth matrix is completed, at around age seven, nature provides that the child functionally separate (through a division of labor in the mind-brain system) from direct dependence on the mother as the base of exploration and shift to the earth itself as the safe place to stand. The earth, structured as a primary knowing structure in the brain, then becomes the source of power and possibility as well. Development then moves toward structuring a knowledge of personal power in interacting with that world matrix.

From the years seven to eleven (roughly), the child structures a knowledge of this personal power in the world. This knowledge of the self (one's mind-brain-body organism) as matrix grows through the child's physical interactions with the physical body of the earth, much as the early infant structured a knowledge of the mother through sensory interactions with her. Dramatic and profound new modes of interaction unfold for development during this late-childhood period. Autonomy—becoming physically independent of parental help and learning to physically survive the principles of the physical world—is the goal of the period. Development of this personal power prepares for a shift of matrix from earth to self.

By adolescence, the biological plan is that we become our own matrix, consisting of mind-brain and body. In the logic of differentiation, mind-brain activity slowly distinguishes from body activity or body-knowing, that concrete knowledge structured throughout childhood. The biological plan then drives us toward the fifth matrix shift, when mind-brain should functionally (through distinctions of brain processing) separate from body. Standing on the matrix of the concretely oriented physical body, mind-brain interactions (pure abstract thinking) should begin matrix formation. That is, the mind-brain should eventually become its own matrix, its own source of power, possibility, and safe place to stand.

At some point after maturity, mind should begin a functional separation, or logical differentiation, from brain processes. This is the final matrix shift that we can have any direct knowledge about. At that point, mind is capable of operating on the structures within its own brain and restructuring its experienced reality accordingly. At that point, personal awareness is no longer contingent upon or dependent upon any concreteness. Thus, the progression from concreteness toward abstraction would be complete.

So long as we live (or she lives), the physical mother remains the primary matrix even though we separate from her and move into larger matrices. Throughout our lives, the earth remains the matrix of all matrices. No matter how abstract our explorations of pure thought and created reality, the mind draws its energy from the brain, which draws its energy from the body matrix, which draws its energy from the earth matrix.

The entire progression can be seen as the growth or development of autonomy, both as a physical organism in the physical world and as a personality in the realm of thought. We have, in effect, only two matrices: the physical matrix, progressing from womb, mother, earth, and physical body, and the abstract matrix of thought, progressing from relationships, the ability for interaction. This interacting ability moved through the physical matrices of womb, mother, earth, body to the abstract matrices of mind-brain with other mind-brains, mind with other minds, and finally, I suppose, mind with "mind-at-large," to use Aldous Huxley's phrase. Separation from any matrix is a birth process, and so we find our entire lives a series of births. This process completes its thrust toward pure abstraction only at death, of course, when all concreteness is transcended, but such remains speculation.[1]

Nature has programmed every conceivable safeguard into the biological plan. The execution of her plan is, sadly, highly problematic and subject to diaster because it can only be built in as *intent*. The success of the plan hinges directly on the infant-child's being provided with a *content* proper for that intent. A proper content is one appropriate to a particular stage of the child's development. The biological plan is wrecked when the intent of nature is met, not with appropriate content, but with the *intentions* of an anxiety-driven parent and culture. Interaction can only take place when content matches intent. Inappropriate content brings about reaction, not intellectual growth. Anxiety results when the child is forced into mismatched relating of intent and content. Interchange with the matrix and growth of personal power then break down, but the sequential unfolding of maturation goes right ahead. The child's ability to interact falls more and more behind, and more and more energy must go into compensation. The young person's intelligence is still back there trying to make the first matrix functional. Finally, there is a breakdown in the mind-brain balance, which was designed to be smoothly synchronous.

When the capacity for abstract creativity and pure thought does not develop properly, the solution is not to try to force earlier and earlier abstract thinking, as we now try to do. Rather, we must provide for full-dimensional interaction with the living earth, without allowing abstract ideas to intercede or obscure, so that a sufficient concrete structure may be built from which abstractions *can* arise.

Our 3-billion-year heritage is truly magnificent; the promise given us is infinite in scope. But this biological plan must be nurtured, and in order to do so, we must first recognize that such a plan exists and then learn something of what that plan is about. We knew about this plan when we were around six years old and a great excitement, longing, and joyful anticipation filled us. Something else happened, of course; and even as it happened, we knew intuitively that it was all wrong. This primary knowing got covered up by anxiety conditioning, which was so deep and pervasive, so ingrained, and so continually reinforced and amplified on every hand that the deep knowing has been lost to us.

The intent of this book is to uncover this knowing in you and to verify and reassure your knowing. We must rekindle our knowing of a personal power that can flow with the power of all things and never be exhausted. We must rekindle a faith in a life system that is our matrix and designed to support us. Only through faith in yourself and in your own life can you respond to a new life given you (either your offspring or your own lost self) according to the needs of that new life.

Paradoxically, for most of us parents, it may only be through response to our children that this faith can be recovered because only the child expresses it openly. We are in a kind of double bind: Only through faith can we open to the life process within us and make a proper response of nurturing our children, and only through that response can we again open to and reclaim our faith and personal power. What we will find is that only by our initial actions, in which we act as though we *had* personal power and knew what to do, can we, in fact, activate that power and knowing. Understanding follows knowing, and knowing results from actions, and proper actions can follow only some deep, intuitive hunch that bypasses ordinary thinking. Our first step is to consider that it just might be possible that nature knew what she was doing when she devised this 3-billion-year developmental plan.

Chapter 3

Intelligence As Interaction

Interaction is a two-way exchange of energy, with an amplification of the energy of each of the two forces. Ordinary *action* is a one-way movement of energy toward or against something. When I chop down a tree, I expend my energy without a corresponding exchange of energy from the tree. Action usually brings about a reaction; the tree falls, and I have to get out of the way. *Reaction* is a one-way movement away from. No exchange and augmenting of energy takes place in either acting or reacting, and we always tire when energy flows out in this way. In true interaction, however, we never tire.

Through interaction, intelligence grows in its ability to interact. We are designed to grow and be strengthened by every event, no matter how mundane or awesome. The flow of nature and seasons, people, extreme contrasts, apparent catastrophes, pleasantries—all are experiences of interaction to be enjoyed and opportunities for learning, leading to greater ability to interact.

With what is human intelligence designed to interact? With anything and everything possible. If there is anything intelligence cannot interact with, that intelligence is to that extent crippled. A fully developed intelligence is one designed to exchange energies with anything existing, without ever being overwhelmed. A mature intelligence should be able to interact on three levels that correspond to and arise from the three stages of biological growth. These levels are: first, the ability to interact with the living earth according to the principles and natural laws of this earth; second, the ability to interact with the earth according to the principles of creative logic developed in the mind-brain system; and third, the ability to interact with the processes and products of the mind-brain system itself, which means the thoughts and creations of our own mind, the minds of others, and the whole thought system underlying our reality. Any definition of intelligence that does not encompass these three categories of interaction is incomplete. Any development of intelligence that does not move through these three modalities falls short of the biological plan for intelligence and betrays nature's 3-billion-year investment and trust.

We have seen how these three ways of interaction are also the three matrices that should form in the developmental years. As adults, we should have three safe places to stand at any time: the earth, our relationships, our own power of thought. And, of course, we should have these safe spaces as sources of possibility from which to choose experience and as sources of energy with which to explore those possibilities.

How should this ability develop? Only by a full development of each of the matrices in the order arranged by the biological plan: developing a knowledge of the world itself, then a knowledge of the creative relations possible with that world, and then a knowledge of creative relations and possibilities themselves. Development can take place only on the foundation given by the child's actual body movements, making sensory contact with the world of things and processes. The growth of intelligence rests on a sensorimotor process, a coordination of the child's muscular system with his/her sensory system and general brain processes.

Any bodily involvement by the early child brings about a patterning in his/her brain system concerning that movement and all the sensory information related to it. For instance, a parent can manipulate the limbs of a newborn infant, and even though they are not initiated by the infant, the bodily movements will in themselves bring about a corresponding pattern of activity in the brain concerning that ability. If repeated sufficiently, these arbitrarily induced puppetlike movements (such as achieving head balance, sitting up, grasping) will lead to that infant's ability to initiate and complete these movements months ahead of an infant who is not so stimulated. The brain patterns for sensorimotor coordinates form automatically.

Intellectual growth is an increase in ability to interact, which means a coordinated flow of the mind-brain-body with the experience at hand. This increase can only take place by the infant-child's interacting with new phenomena. That is, intelligence can only grow by moving from that which is known into that which is not yet known, from the predictable into the unpredictable. The institutionalized child, for instance, does not grow intellectually. Mental retardation is inevitable when the physical environment is unvaried, when new stimuli are almost nonexistent (staring at a gray ceiling or the walls of a crib day and night), and above all, when there is no bodily contact with a stable caretaker to furnish a known matrix. Moving into the unknown is possible only when there is a secure matrix to which the child can make an immediate return, and the younger the child, the more immediate and constant this return must be.

The early child thinks in action and acts his/her thinking. Intellectual growth is a biological process, taking place below awareness as nonconsciously as the growth of hair or teeth. Our conscious awareness is the end product of biological functions. The infant-child learns from every interaction, and all future learning is based on the character of these early, automatic body-brain patterns. This primary sensory organization and response takes precedence over all future learning, even though it never becomes conscious in any ordinary sense. Rather, this base structure furnishes consciousness as well as the possibilities for further learning.

The only criterion we have for what the infant, child, young adult, or adult is learning or has learned is interaction. Can the child or person interact, or is his/her life one long chain of reactions to or acts of aggression against? When people express reaction-aggression, they are expressing not just a crippled intelligence but what they have actually learned.

Growth of the infant-child's ability to interact means increased rhythmic patterning in the brain and corresponding muscular responses. This growth can be slowed almost to a standstill by subjecting the growing child to demands inappropriate to his/her stage of development, that is, by trying to force the child to learn or deal with information or experience suitable to a later stage of development or by keeping them locked into an earlier stage. Then the child learns that learning itself is difficult and frustrating or nonrewarding. Even when the child manages to comply with demands suitable to a later stage, premature involvement can cripple intelligence, although the damage may not show for years.

For instance, abstract knowledge, such as adult idea systems and opinions, is designed for the later years of development. Forcing the early child to deal prematurely with adult abstract thought can cripple the child's ability to think abstractly later on. The first ten years or so are designed for acquiring a full-dimensional knowledge of the world as it is and learning how to interact with it physically and mentally. This growth of knowledge and ability should lead to the ability to survive physically in the world. With the security of a full knowledge of survival, the young person could then move freely into abstract thought. His/her intelligence could then attend the true maturation of the mind-brain. Not incidentally, the concrete knowledge from which survival grows is also the concrete structure of knowledge out of which abstract thought arises.

A shallow-dimensional world view, based only on the long-range senses of sight and sound, is often the kind of knowledge constructed by the child. Direct physical contact with the world—taste, touch, even smell—are often either discouraged or actually forbidden in the parent's anxiety over the hazards of germs and imagined threats. Without a full-dimensional world view structured in the formative years, no earth matrix can form, no knowledge of physical survival can develop, and no basis for abstraction and creativity can arise. A permanent anxiety and obsessive-compulsive attachment to material objects will result. And anxiety always cripples intelligence; it blocks the development of muscular-mindedness, the ability to interact with the unknown and unpredictable. Anxiety is the source of the fall of the child somewhere around age nine. Its roots are deep, its branches prolific, its fruit abundant, and its effects devastating.

Chapter 4

Stress and Learning

Intelligence grows by moving from the known-predictable into the unknown-unpredictable. When we know the probable outcome of an event taking place around us, our body systems can remain fairly passive and relaxed. We can maintain touch with our environment by the skimpiest of sensory samplings; that is, we need attend the world around us only sporadically and peripherally.[1] Our senses bring us a ceaseless stream of reports concerning our world, but these grow humdrum and tedious. A surprising amount of life is repetitious, and after a time, any repetition tends to be screened out of awareness. We shift the editing of repetitive sensory reports to automatic brain processes in order to free our awareness for internal processes of thinking such as daydreaming. We spend a large part of our adult lives establishing routines that allow us to function with a minimum of sensory sampling.

The unknown is a set of circumstances whose outcome we cannot be sure of. The unknown-unpredictable imposes sensory data that do not fit the brain's established editorial policies well enough to be handled automatically by various subordinates. Then the editor in chief, I, the decision-making self must be summoned to the scene. All body processes must be alerted.

The body has an alert mechanism just for the purpose of this coordina-

29

tion. This alert mechanism is activated when sensory data report an event that goes beyond the boundaries of the automatic known-predictable. When this happens, the pituitary gland releases hormones that activate the adrenal steroids. These hormones stimulate and activate the body-brain system in whatever amount the situation seems to call for, whether just a bit to liven up the sleepy system or a massive amount for an all-out frightful emergency.

This organizing of the body and brain to deal with the immediacy of an event and respond accordingly is *stress.* Such an activating and coordinating of the body's muscular system with the sensory system and awareness shuts out imagination and gives a direct sensory involvement, an immediacy that we call *excitement.* The infant is born into the world in a state of general excitement, or stress. Children and young people actively seek out the stress of excitement, often to the despair of their parents. Adults must have some form of excitement-stress, and most of us seek it within the bounds of safety by experiencing it either vicariously, by television, or in mountain climbing, hang-gliding, skiing, tennis, racing, adultery, or what have you.

The average human brain has some 10 billion neurons, or thinking cells, but intelligence rests not so much on the number of cells as on the number of connections between these cells. A neuron can have as many as 10,000 connecting links (dendrites and axons) with other cells or almost none. A single cell can be directly and indirectly linked with as many as 600,000 other cells. These connecting links and the patterns of rhythmic cell firing possible through such linkages are what provide the ability to process information.[2] The more connections, the greater the brain's computational ability.

Stress is the way intelligence grows. At moments of extreme stress, the pituitary gland produces a hormone called *adrenocorticotropic hormone* (ACTH) which, in turn, activates the adrenal steroids, tightening up the body's defense systems. Scientists have injected rats with ACTH and found that the rats immediately produce large quantities of new proteins in the liver and brain. Proteins of this sort seem instrumental in both learning and memory. And on being injected with ACTH, the rat's brain immediately grows massive numbers of new connecting links between the neurons.[3] The same results can be obtained by simply subjecting rats to electric shock for twenty minutes a day. Electric shock creates extreme stress in the rats. The stress brings about ACTH production and the adrenal steroid chain is alerted as the system tries to process the radically threatening sensory information and make an accommodation or adapt to it.

Such stimulated rats prove to be far more intelligent and adaptable than nonstimulated rats. They can learn faster than ordinary rats, solve problems more easily, adapt more quickly, and survive much better. Before converting your high chair to an electric chair, however, bear in mind that although the stressed mind-brain grows in ability and the unstressed one lags behind, the overstressed one collapses into physiological shock and shuts out everything. Stressing the system is only *half* of the natural cycle of learning.

The English scientist Hans Selye won a Nobel Prize for his analysis in *The Stress of Life* (the title of his book on the subject). Selye showed that all life forms are balances of stress and relaxation. Stress-relaxation is a yin-yang effect. You cannot have one without the other if life is to be maintained. Even the elements of physical matter (atoms, molecules, and such) exist in a balance of stress and relaxation.

The rhythm of intellectual growth is movement into the unknown-unpredictable, or stress, and assimilating or digesting it back into the known-predictable, or relaxation. Each such assimilation and adaptation to the unknown increases the scope of the known, the relaxed state. Correspondingly, each such adaptation increases the ability to move into more unknowns, presenting even greater stress or unpredictability, because of the broader base of predictability through which we *can* assimilate the unknown and make a proper accommodation to it.

For most of us, prolonged alertness proves exhausting; after some high-stress encounter, we collapse into a heap of relaxation, generally aided by a few cocktails. Our lives are not a calm balance of the yin and yang of stress and relaxation, in which we remain permanently alert in a relaxed way. They are a wild swing back and forth between anxious tension and sensory retreat.

Coordinating, decision making, rerouting of new sensory data and making new accommodations all require a general alertness or stress equal to the job at hand. Consider, for instance, the many minor emergencies that take place while you drive your car. Once you have learned to drive, the automatic pilot within you can take over and free your general consciousness for daydreaming or talking to yourself or to others while driving. In an emergency, however, you must stop talking and attend to what the automatic pilot was previously attending to. The body's flight-fight response takes control until the emergency is over, and this leaves no part of you for conversation. When an emergency is over, the all-clear sounds in the body, the production of adrenal steroids stops, the heartbeat returns to normal, and the muscles relax. But if the outcome is not successful and stress piles on top of stress, then shock, a condition of sensory cutoff, may occur. When sensory information brings in nothing but waves of high stress and critical danger that we cannot adapt to, the body may shut out all sensory intake.

What the body learns in such a state is negative. It learns that it has survived the high stress by a blackout of reality itself, a minor death.

Failure to assimilate and accommodate to new information breeds the confusion and anxiety of unresolved stress. To enter into an unpredictable situation and accept it openly is to flow with its energy, be augmented in your own energy, and relax its tensions and stresses accordingly.

To interact with a high-stress situation means to have the ability to accept the stress. Ability in this sense is the same as the ability to lift a heavy object or run up a flight of stairs. Stress-relaxation is an ability of the mind-brain, and muscular-mindedness must be developed, just as body musculature must be developed. Intellectual strength is a muscular-mindedness by which greater and more complex unknown-unpredictable situations can be entered into, assimilated by the brain system, and accommodated by a proper response.

The successful intelligence knows, and is able to act on the knowledge, that the life principle of stress-relaxation is inviolate, just as the atom holds its fantastic stresses in a relaxed balance. The strong intelligence knows that stress must create its own relaxation when the natural mind-brain-body process of interaction is allowed to unfold. A developed intelligence is one that knows, and can act accordingly, that no matter how stringent or apparently destructive some opposing force might seem to be, the stress-relaxation principle must hold. By interacting with a force or event, its energy must augment our own and give us power over any destructive elements within that situation.

The weight lifter builds his power through stressing and relaxing his muscles. Muscular-mindedness is built through successful practices of stress-relaxation. This gives personal power and is the source of joy. However, the cycle can take place only from a firm matrix or known base of power, and our job as parents is to make sure that this construction is successful in the infant-child. The genetic plan prepares for, and tries to assure the formation of, just such a secure base of knowing, right from the beginning. The periods of prenatal life, delivery, birth, and infancy are all genetically designed to provide exactly the kinds of experience needed for the brain to structure its place of power.

The mother is the infant's first matrix and the source of his/her possibility. She is the place of power on which the child builds muscular-mindedness and develops autonomy, the self-sufficient strength to separate from her and become independent. If this matrix does not become fully structured, if such a security and strength are not given from birth, intelligence will have no ground on which to grow. The growing intelligence (and, God knows, the so-called mature one) that has no firm matrix has no choice but to devote its energy and attention to trying to secure that matrix. Without that safe place to stand, no energy can be utilized to explore possibility, intent cannot move into content and know fulfillment, and the stress of the unknown-unpredictable becomes a chronic threat. We then spend our lives trying to avoid this threat.

An intelligence whose matrix as mother has not formed sufficiently at birth cannot explore and structure a knowledge of the earth on a full-dimensional level. For this child, the earth as matrix cannot become functional, as designed, when the child is about seven years of age. Rather than the whole world becoming the source of possibility, energy, and the safe place to stand, it becomes the enemy, the adversary, the danger. The person denied the first matrix remains grounded in that earliest stage, trying to establish some arbitrary and artificial safe place of his/her own making. It is a compensation that never works.

Chapter 5

The New Demonology:
Exorcising Nature

The headline of a national newspaper ran: "Stress, the Enemy Within." Medicine men, the article reported, considered stress one of the major killers of our day. In an article on brain research, a prominent magazine featured a medicine man's glowing account of new chemicals by which we could combat stress. By synthetically matching certain body chemicals, we can now fool the body into relaxing its high state of chronic stress. Thus, this medicine man gloated, a chemotherapy pill will replace the (sadly inefficient) psychiatrist or psychologist, and we may all live happily in a state of chemical euphoria.

Stress, of course, is the very fiber of life and surely of intelligence. Why should—indeed, how *did*—stress become the enemy within? Obviously the life-giving balance of stress and relaxation has been seriously upset. We are locked into a cultural stress-stress atmosphere in which relaxation becomes almost impossible unless it is chemically induced. It is stress-stress that truly proves to be the enemy, an alliance with death; but so is relaxation-relaxation because if such a state completely takes over, we must put that body six feet under.

Consider, as a minor example of stress avoidance, our attempts to maintain a constant womb temperature lest we become unpleasantly aware of our bodies, that is, lest our bodies be stressed by hot and cold. Womb temperature has grown to a national obsession, demanding ever greater outputs of personal energy, time, money, and attention to maintain. The procedures of maintenance become more and more stressful, of course, as the enemy to be avoided slowly weaves an inescapable net around us.

To trace the root causes of this notion of stress as the enemy within us would take volumes because it would lead to the unraveling of the whole fabric of current life. I shall focus on only the most significant assumption that underlies this notion and show how it is the real issue before us. This assumption, which really cripples us, is so axiomatic, so much a part of our whole web of beliefs that to question it seems ridiculous. The assumption runs like this: In this 3 billion years of experimenting, life has evolved our huge and brilliant mind-brain system in order that we might have the intelligence to outwit and so survive this life system that has evolved us. That is, we really believe that we have a superior brain in order that we might outwit nature, and we believe we *must* outwit nature in order to survive her. Outwitting means acting against, dominating, overcoming, removing the causes of stress. Interaction, the cooperative flow of energy with the life system, is then quite lost to view.

In Chapter 18, I will show how this notion of outwitting nature literally splits our mind-brain system because it poses one half of the brain as the enemy of the other half and turns what should be a splendid synergy into warring camps. Would a 3-billion-year experiment in genetic coding really have produced as its finest product a brain whose only purpose is to outwit itself? Yet, we believe, apparently with a tenacious passion, that the purpose of human intelligence is to predict and dominate the infinitely contingent and interacting balances of a universal system. We call our supposed successes in this venture *progress* and believe that the purpose of our lives is to contribute to this progress. Finally, we gauge all our interpretations of intelligence according to this belief, at which point we surely fall—long and hard.

How do we believe that we can predict and control the natural forces of the universe? Through clever intellectual manipulations and tool usage. We accept this notion so completely because we have been conditioned to believe implicitly that only by so using our intelligence can we, in fact, survive nature. Interaction between the mind-brain and its source of information has been rigorously, religiously denied by Western logic, if not *most* cultural logic. Interaction with the living earth would imply that the earth responded in kind, interacting with us. And the one cardinal rule of all classical Western academic belief, which is very much in power over our minds today, is that the mind has absolutely no relation to the world other than to be informed of that world through the senses and to make some sort of intelligent reaction to that information. This belief has automatically robbed us of personal power. Having no personal power to draw on, we are reduced to only one source of power: tool usage. And so, we have evolved a continuing body of knowledge concerning the employment, creation, enhancement, and service of tools. Our real criterion of value becomes the culture's body of knowledge offering or promising enhanced tool production, possible domination of nature, and so some security. Potential is seen as an increase of tools. The training and education of children is designed to lead to better tool invention, production, consumption, and handling.

Our body of knowledge and tool development has never given, is not presently giving, and almost surely will never give us either physical security or well-being. The more vast and awesome our tool production has become, the greater our anxiety, hostility, fear, resentment, and aggression. But the direct correlation between our anxiety and tool production is almost beyond our grasp because our intelligence is itself the result of our conditioning by and within that very body of knowledge. Our intelligence is trained to believe that any imperfections in the reality resulting from our activities, such as personal anguish, misery, and fear, simply indicates the need for improvements in the body of knowledge and/or improvements in tool production, distribution, and application. Even as our body of knowledge splits us off from our lives and creates anxiety and unhappiness, it conditions us to believe religiously that escape from our misery lies in perfecting that body of knowledge. (Therein lies the current generation's sincere belief in schooling as the way out of our dark ages.)

European and American researchers have long observed that infants do not smile until some two and a half months after birth (on the average). Nor does the early infant display sensorimotor learning or general adaptations during this time. Because such a prolonged period of incapacity, with no signs of intelligence being manifested, is quite unique in this world, many learned papers have been written about the smiling syndrome and postbirth lack of intellectual response in infants. Freud, in early neurological studies of infants, wrote about this strange vegetative condition, and theories have grown out of his theory in typical academic style. Our body of knowledge finally included as a matter of fact that babies do not (indeed perhaps should not) smile during this ten- to twelve-week period after birth because intelligence is nonexistent during this time.

In 1932, Katherine Bridges noted that the newborn seems to come into the world in a state of "general excitement" but that this excitement quickly changes to distress. Pleasure or smiling, she observed, appears some two and a half to three months later. Rene Spitz wrote about the smiling syndrome and its late appearance signaling the beginnings of some crude intelligence. The infant has only two states in this period, he observed, "quiescence," which meant unconsciousness or sleep, and "unpleasure," which meant being awake. Spitz noted that for the first two and a half to three months, the infant either cries or sleeps and little else. Spitz based his position on "Freud's concept of the neonate as a psychologically undifferentiated organism. . . . This organism still lacks consciousness, perception, sensation, and all other psychological functions." At another point, Spitz writes: "I follow Freud's opinion that at birth there is no consciousness, accordingly, there can be no awareness or conscious experience. . . . Thus it is rare to find the smiling response before the third month of life."

Burton White, of Harvard's center for child development, found research futile for about the first two months of life because the infant only sleeps, cries, or feeds during this time. Until smiling begins, he maintained, there is no intelligence.

The question arose: Why is intelligence so slow in forming? No other species has anything comparable to this long delay in at least some form of intelligent adaptation. In answer, theories arose, of course, giving rise to other theories, concerning this period of stupor, total helplessness, semiconsciousness, massive sleeping, excessive crying, and a generally precarious hold on life. Spitz, in fact, assumed that the entire first year of life was devoted solely to physical survival.

Naturally, an acceptable answer emerged: The human infant is born *prematurely*. We are rather like marsupials without pouches. And naturally another question arose: Why is the human born prematurely? Again, an answer dutifully emerged, one in keeping with the whole fallacy. We are born prematurely because of our big brains. Notice that the head of the infant at birth is much larger than the body. Problems arose when humankind got up on its hind legs and started walking upright because this posture closed in the pelvic area and narrowed the birth canal considerably. With this huge head, full of all those brains, if the infant were to grow to full term in utero, his head would be too large to pass through the now-narrowed canal, so the human infant must be born prematurely to get out at all.

No less a person than Jerome Bruner of Harvard's Center for Cognitive Studies, surely one of our more brilliant researchers, developed this idea. The assumption is terribly wrong, but the academic rationale growing around it began to include more contradictions blithely ignored because once an idea is accepted into the body of knowledge, everyone "knows" and no one questions it. Everyone "knew" that no smiling occurs for some ten to twelve weeks because infants are born prematurely and have no intelligence during that time. If a mother reported some smiling before that acceptable date, the cryptic diagnosis was "gas pains."

Meanwhile, in 1956, Marcelle Geber, under a research grant from the United Nations Children's Fund, traveled to Africa to study the effects of malnutrition on infant and child intelligence. She concentrated on Kenya and Uganda and made a momentous discovery. She found the most precocious, brilliant, and advanced infants and children ever observed anywhere. These infants had smiled, continuously and rapturously, from, at the latest, their fourth day of life. Blood analyses showed that all the adrenal steroids connected with birth stress were totally absent by that fourth day after birth. Sensorimotor learning and general development were phenomenal, indeed miraculous. These Ugandan infants were months ahead of American or European children. A superior intellectual development held for the first four years of life. (Why it ended there will be a point of study in Chapter 7.)

These infants were born in the home, generally delivered by the mother herself. The child was never separated from the mother, who massaged, caressed, sang to, and fondled her infant continually. The mother carried her unswaddled infant in a sling, next to her bare breasts, continually. She slept with her infant. The infant fed continuously, according to its own schedule. These infants were awake a surprising amount of the time—alert, watchful, happy, calm. They virtually never cried. Their mothers were bonded to them (an issue I shall discuss more thoroughly in Chapter 7) and sensed their every need before that need had to be expressed by crying. The mother responded to the infant's every gesture and assisted the child in any and every move that was undertaken, so that every move initiated by the child ended in immediate success. At two days of age (forty-eight hours) these infants sat bolt upright, held only by the forearms, with a beautifully straight back and perfect head balance, their finely focused eyes staring intently, intelligently at their mothers. And they smiled and smiled.

New European-type hospitals were being erected in Uganda at the time of Geber's studies (she was granted an additional year to make long-term studies to which I shall return in Chapter 7). Only the upper-class Ugandan families could afford such luxury, of course, and the women of this class naturally followed the fashion of having their children in hospitals. These hospital-delivered infants, it turned out, followed the same civilized schedule American and European infants do. Geber found that they did not smile until some two and a half months after birth. Nor were they precocious in any sense. They showed no signs of sensorimotor learning, displayed no uncanny intelligence for some two and half months, at which point some signs of intelligence were apparent. Blood analyses showed that high levels of adrenal steroids connected with birth stress were still prevalent at two and a half months. These infants slept massively, cried when awake, were irritable and colicky, frail and helpless. So the issue was not in some racial predisposition toward early intellectual growth. The issue lay solely with what happens to the newborn infant in hospitals.

What happens is quite simple: The infant is exposed to an intelligence determined to outwit nature, an intelligence distrustful of anything natural, an intelligence with a vast array of tools at its disposal with which to outwit and, in fact, supplant nature entirely. And in that outwitting and supplanting, damage is done that is incalculable. Future historians will shudder in loathing and horror at the hospital treatment of newborns and mothers in this very dark age of the medicine man and the surgeon and their uses of chemicals and cuttings. The chemicals dull and stupefy both mother and infant, making birth hazardous, prolonged, difficult, and extreme; so tools are used for grappling, clawing, sucking the infant out when the natural processes have been made impossible.[1]

The Ugandan mother works around her house until some five minutes before delivery. In about an hour, she is out on the streets again, showing her new infant to her neighbors and relatives.

Frederick LeBoyer was a conventional French obstetrician who delivered 9,000 babies by standard methods. He noticed that France, a nation of 50 million persons, had over 1 million dysfunctional children. He began to question general birth practices and realized that hospital deliveries were damaging the infants. He quit his practice, retired to India for three years, where he carefully studied native procedures for child delivery in very remote, so-called primitive areas. He combined what he saw with his own scientific background and came up with a synthesis. He returned to France and began a new form of delivering infants into the world. And the babies he delivers *smile,* beautifully, continuously, rapturously, from some twelve hours after birth.

I personally know of several infants, delivered in the home by their own parents, who have smiled continuously from the first hour of life. And why not? They have been met with love, care, concern, and above all, gentleness and quiet.

In Chapters 6 and 7, I will show how technological childbirth and conventional Western notions about the treatment of infants produce an infant who can show no signs of intelligence and surely no signs of pleasure for those standard two and a half months. I will show that the aftereffects of technological hospital delivery are permanent. We have built an elaborate body of knowledge not only rationalizing the damage we have done, but also accepting the damaged product as natural and inevitable. And we accept all the massive problems resulting as "human nature."

As a father of five children, my first reaction to the evidence gathering about me was to shut it out. I did not want to know. I had done the best I could, as had my wife. We had acted conscientiously to a painful degree. We had no recourse but to accept the words of the authorities, for we were products of the age of professionalism. And it has taken me a long while to realize that we were not guilty, a point I want to emphasize here for other parents caught as we were.

Chapter 6

Time Bomb:
In the Delivery Room

All the anxiety-ridden fallacies of our day seem to congregate in the hospital delivery room, where they bring about a disaster that remains largely undetected because it works like a time bomb. None of the parties to the crime ever has to pay, for the explosion takes place in slow fusion over the years and creates such widespread and diverse havoc that few bother to trace it back to see who lit the fuse.

The fallacies are personified in the figure of the medicine man, who, donning his bizarre and frightful masks and cloaks and surrounded by an astonishing array of mechanical wizardry, sets about to outwit nature. Aided by an equally impressive array of chemicals, he sets about to help the victim-patient-mother avoid the stress inherent within the strange unfolding nightmare. Lost to sight, almost incidental and peripheral to the play of ego, money, and power involved, is the the infant, the new life trying to unfold. As everyone "knows," this psychologically undifferentiated organism lacks consciousness, perception, sensation, and all other psychological functions. Accordingly, there can be no awareness. So the attitude is: Get the infant out of the way quickly so that we adults can enjoy our self-drama.

At what point does intelligence, the interaction between an organism and its environment, begin to function? All development, physical and mental, seems to follow a *cycle of competence*, to use Greenfield and Tronick's term.

First, there is a roughing in of raw materials, the accumulation of a certain critical mass sufficient to work with. Then, there is the filling in of details, an ordering and structuring of that raw mass. Finally, there is a practice of the resulting possibility and an exploration of the variables it affords.

Somewhere between the eighth and twelfth weeks of fetal development, brain growth begins in an explosion of activity, far outstripping body growth. The growth of brain cells is a hodgepodge at this early stage. There is a wild profusion of all the different types of cells: those of the high roof brain, those of the basal ganglia, and those to be used for vision, hearing, or in the cerebellum. All these are mixed together without apparent rhyme or reason other than multiplication. This is the period of roughing in. We could hardly call this kind of a growth an organism, much less a thinking organism, because it has no organization. Or has it?

Whenever any two like cells are in proximity, they tend to function as a unit. Place two living heart cells a distance apart on a microscopic slide and watch them. They will pulsate randomly, each at its own rate. Move these cells closer together, and at some critical point (they do not have to touch), they will arc the gap between, somehow communicate with each other, and begin to pulsate together and function as a heart. So almost surely, even two brain cells in proximity begin some preliminary form of interaction. This may not rate as *thought* in any mature sense, but there is almost surely a form of learning taking place.[1]

Around the fifth prenatal month, this roughing in of raw materials achieves its critical mass, and the cycle of competence shifts to filling in the details. A "mysterious signal," as Sperry calls it, fires into this randomness, and a marvelous ordering instantly begins to take place. With a rush, the cells begin to differentiate and organize themselves according to their innate functions. Neural cells of the optical type start lining themselves into nerves to carry messages from the eyes; aural cells, to carry messages from the ears; cerebellum cells, to group themselves into that coherent organ next to the old brain.

From this point on, the brain functions as a brain, and the function of the brain is to learn. The driving intent within is always to interact with, and learn of, the content without and to gain the abilities of that interaction. Thinking must automatically take place once a thinking organ organizes. To speak of a living being or conscious organism for the first five months in the womb may be a matter of aesthetics, but not to recognize the infant in utero as a living, responsive, intelligent creature after that fifth month is ignorance, a blatant ignoring of evidence.

Because the research on this subject has grown to such massive proportions in recent years, I will confine my example to one aspect of infant intelligence (and relegate additional evidence to the Notes and Bibliography).[2] Language has long been considered the most difficult, sophisticated, and complex learning the mind-brain has achieved. The resulting debate among linguists has long been: How can the child learn language as rapidly as s/he does? After all, language is simply too complex to be so rapidly assimilated. (By about age four, the child's linguistic structure is complete, lacking only logical refinement and vocabulary extension.) Noam Chomsky, of MIT, for instance, proposed that language must be in some way innate, built into the genes, a proposal that has drawn much ire and fire from all around.

Back in the 1940s, Bernard and Sontag found that the infant in utero immediately responded with body movements to sounds from the mother and to sounds in her immediate environment. In 1970, Brody and Axelrod stated categorically that there were no *random* movements in the newborn infant or in the uterine infant. Every movement, they insisted, has meaning, purpose, and design. (Within minutes after birth, the newborn begins, in his wake state, almost continuous movement of his limbs, body, and head.)

In 1974, two Boston University researchers, Doctors William F. Condon and Louis Sander, published a study on the so-called random movements observable in newborn infants. Through sophisticated analysis of high-speed sound movies of scores of newborn infants, Condon and Sander found that these so-called random movements immediately coordinated with speech when speech was used around the infants.[3] Computer studies further revealed that each infant had a complete and individual repertoire of body movements that synchronized with speech; that is, each infant had a specific muscular response to each and every part of his/her culture's speech pattern. One infant, for instance, might move his/her left elbow slightly every time a *k* sound (as in *cough* or *cat*) was used. The sound *ah* (as in *father*) might elicit a movement of the right foot or perhaps the big toe. These movements proved consistent; the infant made the same movement to the same sound or sequence of sounds.

Condon and Sander found that they could catalog and computerize an infant's repertoire of movement coordinates, make up an artificial sound tape of random speech parts, and feed this to the computer to match the tape to the infant's personal repertoire. The computer would then predict the precise movements the infant would make to each of the sounds as they played. Condon and Sander would then play the tape to the infant, making their high-speed movies as they did so. They then checked the results frame by frame; inevitably, each sound produced the matching physical movement as computerized and cataloged.

They then studied older children and finally adults and found the patterns of synchronization to be universal and permanent. By adulthood, the movements have become microkinetic, discernible only by instrumentation, but nevertheless clearly detectable and invariant. The only exception found was in autistic children, who exhibited no such body-speech patterning (a point that sorely needs to be considered by those persons and institutions working with autistic children).

Because the newborn infant has a distinct repertoire of movements (each child's is unique) and the synchronicity can be observed within some twelve minutes after birth, logic almost compels us to accept as fact that the infant has structured this patterned response or surely at least roughed in the patterns while in the womb. Certainly, the drive for this patterning must be considered innate, part of that driving *intent* within needing only the content from without to interact with. Intent preceding the ability to *do* is the key here. Actual speech does not appear until about a year after birth, but nature has prepared for that momentous and awesome capacity long before.

My point in this example is that *learning* is taking place in utero, and it is a learning of the most complex and intricate human structure. That a learning of such dimensions begins in utero compels us to reevaluate our notions of learning, perhaps of speech itself, and surely our notions about the infant as a "nondifferentiated psychic organism."

The Condon-Sander study also indicates the thorough and awesome reaches of nature's biological plan, and we must seriously reexamine our notions and ideas about childbirth and treatment of the newborn. Perhaps now you can see why my statements about the infant in utero structuring a knowledge of his first matrix-world were not at all fanciful. For that is exactly what takes place in those last months of prenatal life—or, rather, what *should* take place.

When the proper gestation period is over, and the infant is ready to leave his/her first matrix and embark on the great venture into the world, it is *his/her* body that releases the hormones triggering the entire birth-delivery system. The mother's body picks up the hormones released by the infant, which, in turn, trigger her hormones into action. These hormones are passed back to the infant, and back and forth it goes. The two systems, mother's and child's, are designed to work together for a quick, efficient delivery. The birth canal is, after all, very short.

Intelligence grows by moving from the known to the unknown and referring back to the known. And never again in life, perhaps not even in death, will intelligence have to make such an extreme and sudden movement, adaptation, and learning, in so short a time as that involved in being born into this world. The environmental change is the most extreme that will ever be experienced; the known bears so few points of similarity to the unknown.

Not the least of the extremities of change is the transition of oxygen supply, originally given by the mother's body through the placenta and umbilical cord, to the infant's own lungs. The lungs require about five minutes to begin functioning and establish sufficient regularity. Once this is established, the heart shuts off that valve shunting blood through the umbilical cord to the placenta and directs the total blood supply through the lungs. For this critical transition period, nature has provided the infant with a fail-safe mechanism because even a short time of oxygen deprivation permanently damages the brain. (The brain gulps oxygen at a prodigious rate, consuming more than the rest of the body.) The placenta contains some 30 percent of the infant's blood and oxygen supply in reserve to cover this transition, and nature provides some twenty-six inches of umbilical cord so that the infant can remain in contact with this reserve supply even after his/her passage. The cord is just the right length, in fact, to allow the infant to be clasped to his/her mother's breast without breaking the connection with his/her oxygen reserves.

Birth is a potential trauma for the infant even when all goes well. (And we must remind ourselves that this infant is highly intelligent, responsive, busily structuring knowledge, with a brain system five times larger, in size ratio, than his body.) Anoxia, a fear of oxygen deprivation, is a primal terror in us all, bringing on a flight-fight alert of major proportions, and violent change of external conditions is something that we seem to try to avoid at all costs.

Following its shifts of position to align properly with the birth canal, the infant's body prepares for delivery by releasing certain hormones. First in line is that master hormone ACTH. ACTH, as we know, brings about large increases of proteins in the liver and brain that are vital to new learning and a corresponding massive growth of new brain-cell connections. At every such influx of new cell connections, the brain is prepared for massive new learnings designed to take place *stage-specifically* (within a designated time span).

The infant's body also releases large amounts of adrenal steroids, those flight-fight arousal hormones that we release when seriously startled or frightened. This adrenal response is the infant's way of organizing his/her entire body for its greatest survival maneuver. Its body assumes a typical flight-fight posture that neatly streamlines it for passage through the canal: toes pointed back, fists clenched, back arched. (These, by the way, are the physical postures many autistic children are locked into permanently.)

This condition of all-out arousal is termed *birth stress.* This condition, with its easily recognized physical manifestations and blood changes, proved a key in Marcelle Geber's (and Mary Ainsworth's) comparative studies of American-European and Ugandan infants. Researchers have long debated the extremes of the infant's stress at birth because the extremity does not seem warranted by the situation. In Chapter 7, I will discuss why the infants *we* see are in such extremities of stress; here, let me give at least three reasons for birth stress in general: First, the physical passage itself, although short in distance and designed by nature to be very short in time, is nevertheless traumatic and not without hazards. The immediate imperative of oxygen production demands extreme alertness of the infant body and total efficiency of all its operations. Adrenalin is just such a stimulant. Second, high stress in the newborn proves to be a key to the physical establishment of *bonding* with the mother (the subject of Chapter 7). Third, and sadly not recognized, birth stress prepares the brain and body for massive new learning. A general alertness, new brain connections, and new proteins are provided for the greatest movement from the known to unknown ever to be undertaken. These three effects prove intricately, intimately interconnected; each depends on the success of the other for its proper fulfillment.

So we have, at the completion of the uterine period, an infant whom nature has prepared for rapid and extensive new learning. First, it must learn to use new bodily processes never used before, which (because of the nature of the womb) cannot be practiced in advance. Second, it must learn a radically different matrix environment, the relationships inherent within that new environment, and the new uses of the body and senses within it. In the outside world, the sensory system is called upon to perform functions radically different from those in utero, and nature depends on specific physical responses from the mother to activate and bring this into play. And nature has programmed into her instinctive physical responses to the infant to meet these highly specific needs. These physical responses not only complete the transition from inter- to extrauterine life but also are a key part of bonding between the mother and infant, on which all development hinges.

And what of the act of birth itself? That act, to put it mildly, varies according to one's culture. When the Australian aborigine mother is ready to deliver, she drops back from her tribe, alone. She digs a hole in the sand, squats over it, delivers her infant, waits for the placenta to discharge, catches and eats the placenta (which is more nourishing than liver and ideal for the mother at that moment, a practice followed by many economical cultures, such as the Eskimo), puts the infant to her breast, and runs to rejoin her tribe. She is gone an average of twenty minutes.

The Ugandan mother, as is typical in nontechnological cultures, follows her usual routines until some five minutes before the baby appears. She retires to a place of privacy, squats, delivers her young (perhaps with help from a midwife, perhaps not), and resumes her ordinary routines within the hour.

The United States has the most expensive medical system in the world and makes childbirth a major economic crisis, for in this country, virtually all children are born in hospitals. The United States also has an astonishingly high infant mortality rate. Not only do our babies die at a record rate (a few years back we stood sixteenth on the list, but we have now pulled ourselves up to thirteenth—a little better than East Germany but not quite up to Hong Kong) but also so do our mothers. As one front-page newspaper story put it: The pill might be dangerous, but it's a lot safer than having a baby. To this, I would add: in the United States, yes.

Holland, where most childbirth takes place in the home with only a midwife in attendance (although ample backup emergency service is ready), had the lowest infant mortality rate in the world (among technological nations, which keep tab on this sort of thing) until Sweden recently took top honors.

In America, birth has become a technological, profit-making event. Pregnancy is quite literally treated as a disease, with technological-surgical delivery the final remedy of that disease. Failure to submit to the medical machinations for childbirth can result in criminal negligence charges or prosecution for practicing medicine (healing the disease of pregnancy) without a license. At an average cost of $1,000 to have a baby in this country, as of this writing ($1,500 for a really first-class delivery, $500 for the cheapie, quickie, God-help-you ghetto delivery) and millions of infants being born yearly, a lot of cold cash is at stake, along with a massive investment of ego and power.

The resistance of the medical people to natural childbirth is understandable. Resistance is displayed to anything natural. The natural does not pay and does not need the professional, who robs you of what is naturally yours and sells it back to you at a dear price. Childbirth as a natural, euphoric, and ecstatic experience—as reported by primitives, hippies who birth in their own dirty homes, or other uncivilized specimens—obviously will not do. Childbirth is, and will damned well be *kept*, dangerous, difficult, painful, complicated, obscure, mysterious, and vastly beyond the grasp of a simple *layperson* (someone who does not even know Latin anatomical terminology). How could women be kept frightened enough to jump through those medical hoops, assume that unnatural position, submit to the series of insults and violations of person and child, and keep those husbands shucking out all those bucks if such a notion as natural childbirth were to take hold?

An apparently incidental issue here, which actually turns out to be monumental, is the position medicine men of the West have, since the time of Louis XIV, forced their victims to take: the *supine* position—flayed out flat on the back and, in a shocking number of cases, even *strapped down,* a position that would strike terror into the staunchest soul.[4] What does the word *supine* mean? Helpless and incompetent. This position throws every muscle and bone of the body completely out of line for natural delivery of an infant from the womb and makes that delivery extremely difficult.

A number of years ago, a doctor by the name of William F. Windle became concerned over childbirth practices. He made a careful analysis of hospital deliveries throughout the United States and noted, with some alarm, two questionable procedures: the widespread, automatic use of premedication and anesthetics and the usual practice of cutting the umbilical cord as soon as the baby's body was clear. There has never been a textbook on obstetrics that did not stress leaving the umbilical cord strictly alone so long as any activity is detectable in it. How and why this strict injunction got so completely lost in medical practice is too involved to discuss here. Suffice it to say that Windle's observations proved to be too tragically accurate; the umbilical cord is cut almost immediately in the majority of cases.[5]

Windle then made the simplest of tests. He took pregnant monkeys and treated them to all the benefits of our modern medical practices. At the time of labor and delivery, he administered anesthetics in a body-weight ratio equivalent of that given the average laboring human mother in the hospital. At the birth of the infant, he cut the umbilical cord at the average time he had found practiced in hospitals. In every case, Windle's newborn monkeys could not get their breath and had to be resuscitated; that is, artificial means had to be used to help them get their breath going. (Our hospitals now have various machines to aid in this process.)

In the natural world, of course, this never takes place. Unless an animal infant is stillborn, it breathes the instant that its head clears the cervix. Little monkeys have enormous capability soon after birth. Almost immediately, they can cling to their mother, who resumes her ordinary life quickly, toting her infant with her, giving him a bit of assistance in those first few hours as he clings to her. In a short time, the infant is physically autonomous, on his feet, jumping about, leaping away from his mother and back to her.

Windle's infant monkeys, whose nature had been outwitted by clever human devices, showed no such agility or ability. Indeed, they were totally helpless. Not only could they not cling to the mother, they could not get their limbs under them at all. The mothers, dazed by the drugs and the greatly lengthened labor (which anesthetics automatically cause), could do little to assist.[6] Windle had to step in to keep the little creatures alive. And how long was it before these medically delivered infants achieved some normality, got their limbs under them, and began some preliminary sensorimotor learning? Some two to three weeks.

Windle performed autopsies on some of these helpless infants and found in every case that their brains harbored severe lesions of a type resulting from oxygen deprivation. He was able to keep some of the monkeys alive (and it took outside help; it was beyond the monkeys' abilities) until they had matured and achieved apparent normality. When Windle autopsied some of these apparently recovered monkeys, he found that their brains *still* harbored exactly the same lesions found at birth. The damage done at the beginning proved irreparable.

Windle next studied human infants who had died following known birth histories of anesthetics, low Apgar scoring, premature cutting of the umbilical cord, and so on. Autopsies showed that these infant brains harbored exactly the same lesions he had found in his oxygen-deprived monkeys. Cases of children who had similar birth histories but who died at age three or four were then studied, and where possible, autopsies were made. Again, the brains were found with the same lesions.

Windle pointed out the obvious. In those first critical moments when the lungs must make the transition to producing all the oxygen for that young body, the system expects to call on the reserve supply held in the placenta. A drugged mother immediately means a drugged infant, and a drugged infant cannot get his/her breath. Artificial means must be used. Breathing is then clumsy, slow, inefficient. The cutting of the umbilical cord at this time denies the infant the reserves of oxygen at the most critical point in his/her life. A vicious double bind is imposed.

Windle found that the majority of hospital deliveries required resuscitation. Now, what is the most familiar birth scene that comes to your mind? What do we think of as a universal, natural part of childbirth? Spanking the baby. Holding the newborn up by the heels and vigorously belting him/her on the backside in the hope that air will get going in that tired, drugged system. This is resuscitation. These infants failed to breathe (or in many cases, the impatient doctor could not wait or could not stand to stand around waiting), and artificial means had to be used. Nowhere else in nature is failure to breathe noted except in stillborns. And nowhere else do we find this deadly syndrome except in technological, medical, hospital deliveries.

Newell Kephart, director of the Achievement Center for Children at Purdue University, finds learning and behavior problems resulting from minor undetected brain injury in 15 to 20 percent of all children examined. Goldberg and Schiffman estimate that 20 to 40 percent of our school population is handicapped by learning problems that may be related to "neurological impairments at birth."[7]

Windle closed his report, published in *Scientific American* in 1969, with this comment:

> [Our experiments] have taught us that birth asphyxia lasting long enough to make resuscitation necessary always damages the brain. . . . A great many human infants have to be resuscitated at birth. We assume that their brains, too, have been damaged. There is reason to believe that the number of human beings in the U.S. with minimal brain damage due to asphyxia at birth is much larger than has been thought. Perhaps it is time to reexamine current practices of childbirth with a view to avoiding conditions that give rise to asphyxia.

Chapter 7

Breaking the Bond:
Our End Is in Our Beginning;
Our Beginning Is Our End

Jean MacKellar told me of her years in Uganda, where her husband practiced medicine.[1] Local mothers brought their infants to see the doctor, often standing patiently in line for hours. The women carried the tiny infants in a sling, next to their bare breasts. Older infants were carried on the back, papoose style. The infants were never swaddled, nor were diapers used. Yet none of them were soiled when finally examined by the doctor. Puzzled by this, Jean finally asked some of the women how they managed to keep their babies so clean without diapers and such. "Oh," the women answered, "we just go to the bushes." Well, Jean countered, how did they know when the infant needed to go to the bushes? The women were astonished at her question. "How do *you* know when *you* have to go?" they exclaimed.

Konner, in his studies of the Zhun/Twasi, an African hunting-gathering culture, found the infants carried in the Ugandan fashion.[2] These mothers always knew when the infant was going to urinate or defecate and removed the child to the bushes ahead of time. The mother sensed the general state of the infant and anticipated the infant's every need.

These mothers and infants have *bonded. Bonding* is a nonverbal form of psychological communication, an intuitive rapport that operates outside of or beyond ordinary rational, linear ways of thinking and perceiving. Bonding involves what I call *primary processing,* a biological function of enormous practical value, yet largely lost to technological man.

Marshall Klaus of Case Western Reserve Hospital in Cleveland, Ohio, has made the most articulate, thorough, and brilliant study of bonding to date. He has shown how bonding is a carefully programmed instinctual response built into us genetically. The mother is genetically programmed to bond to the infant at his/her birth, and the infant is programmed to expect her response. Indeed, without it, the infant is in grave trouble. Bonding may even involve specific hormones, and breast-feeding may prove one of the most critical factors in establishing the bond.

Carl Jung once said that the child lives in the unconscious of the parent. I am distrustful of the word *unconscious,* but surely Jung was correct about the function involved. The truth is, the fully conscious parent encompasses the psychological state of the child. They participate in shared functions that need no articulation, that simply call for spontaneous response, a mutual meeting of needs and a mutual fulfillment on emotional-intuitive levels.

Bruno Bettleheim pointed out that the early infant never feels helpless so long as his crying can elicit attention and bring about some response from his world. Studies of infantile autism show that as an infant, the autistic child almost never cried or quickly learned never to cry. (And the autistic child never cries again.) Crying seems to be a distress signal employed when other signals fail. If this final form of communication consistently fails to bring response from the caretaker, the infant then learns that it has no power over its world at all and sinks into apathy.

Blurton Jones, in England, points out that the breast-fed infant cries more than the bottle-fed infant, but only during the first year of life. Thereafter, the breast-fed infant cries far *less* than the bottle-fed one. The reason is not hard to find. Breast-feeding automatically establishes some bonds. The breast-feeding mother is more solicitous of the infant's welfare and needs and responds more readily to its cries. The mother who bottle-feeds is automatically operating out of a different attitude; lacking the intimacy of breast-feeding, she is less responsive. She schedules attention and tends not to break that schedule. Her infant finds that his/her crying brings scant results. However, after the first stage of autonomy, somewhere after twelve months or so, when the infant-child can move around and begin to assert him/herself, crying takes on serious proportions, growing into a constant harangue over dissatisfaction and a substitute for personal power. But the breast-fed infant, who found that his/her crying always elicited response from the world, develops some concept of personal power in that world. After the first stage of autonomy, with the additional tools of walking, grasping, climbing, reaching, talking, unfolding, his/her conviction of personal power then extends to these more mature methods of expression. Then crying is used only in emergencies.

Klaus, however, makes the astonishing claim that if properly bonded with the mother, the child should *never* cry. Crying, he states, is an unnatural, abnormal, uncommunicative expression, an emergency distress mechanism only. And in those societies where bonding is practiced, crying is, indeed, quite rare. Other forms of communication are used, and the infants and children develop the sense of personal power such responsiveness gives. Thus, the Ugandan children are (at least *were*) calm, happy, alert, and enormously intelligent. They have a matrix from which to operate.

Given a choice of life companions, I would take any number of brain-damaged people, rather than one unbonded person, for we are flexible beyond measure and can compensate for extensive physical damage, but lack of bonding finds no compensation. Bonding is stage-specific. Nature has designed the bonds to be established in the hours immediately following birth. The preparations have been made far in advance, but, as in the case of learning to breathe, there is a critical period for bonding.

Robert L. Fantz found that newborns could focus on and recognize a human face. His findings, at first widely disputed, were later verified by Klaus. Klaus pointed out, however, that this face-recognition ability was stage-specific to the period immediately after birth. For a short period, the newborn can not only focus on and recognize his/her mother's face but also follow her visually when she moves about the room. The qualifications are —and this is so obvious, yet devastating in implication—that the infant must be undrugged and undamaged, and this innate brain pattern must be *given* that face to focus on if the patterns are to be fully activated. If furnished with the stimuli to bring that pattern into play, the infant will spend some 80 percent of his/her waking time locked in on that face. The brain's pattern for organizing that visual data will thus be strengthened. If not brought into play and continually stimulated, that brain function will quickly disappear, not to be regained for days or weeks.

Face recognition is only one of the many interlocking aspects of bonding. Blind children can bond to the parent. Nevertheless, it plays an essential role in the structure of knowledge of the new matrix, the mother, that the normal infant must build. Establishing this face pattern gives the cornerstone on which the whole conceptual set is built after birth, the constellate around which all the rest of the infant's explorations of the mother will orient.

The newborn knows his/her mother's body odors and distinguishes her voice from any other. After all, s/he has heard that voice throughout the last months in utero. There are numerous other primary sensings of the mother that we have not yet articulated and may never be fully able to. Breast milk may well carry hormones vital to, and supportive of, bonding. The whole thrust is to establish for the newborn a matrix, a sense of security, and a point of reference for the unfolding sensory system and experience.

The issue is not sweet sentiment. The issue is intelligence, the brain's ability to process sensory information, organize muscular responses, and interact with the environment. In order to be assimilated and accommodated by the mind-brain, the unknown experience must have a sufficient number of points of similarity to the known. This is the cycle of stress-relaxation involved in all learning. If there is no way of relating the new to the old, the brain cannot process that information. Confusion and anxiety must then result, and the learning must prove negative.

In the animal world, if a newborn infant is separated from its mother for any length of time, the mother will not recognize the infant when it is returned and may refuse to nurture it. If the infant is separated at birth and kept separate for more than a few hours, it will probably not survive.

All animal mothers (of the higher species, except perhaps some marsupials) lick their newborn offspring thoroughly all over—and not just lightly or just once. This prolonged and thorough licking activates and brings into full function the sensory system of that creature.

Life in the womb calls for a limited use of the sensory system because the creature is floating in a fluid that quite insulates the skin. The human infant, for instance, is coated with a fatty, mucilaginous substance (called *vernix caseosa*) at birth, which actually seems to protect the skin from its constant water immersion in the womb. Therefore, at birth, the sensory system of the infant's body, particularly the myriad nerve endings in the skin, is in a dormant state. But life in the outside world calls for activation of this far-flung nerve apparatus. There is only one way this system can be activated: by being brought to life. How do you bring to life the sense of touch? Only by touching. Just as the visual pattern of face recognition must be activated by being furnished with the stimuli appropriate to it, the other sensory systems must be given appropriate stimuli.

In the midbrain, there is a small area called the *reticular formation.* (This area rises and falls in its popularity for brain research, and after a period on the wane, it is again receiving considerable attention.) Apparently, the body's sensory information is channeled at the reticular formation and dispensed to the various portions of the brain according to the particular kind of information and the area of the brain concentrating on it. The on-off switch for general consciousness, sleep and wake, and such seems to be related to this area.

There is a particular area on a newborn kitten's belly that the mother cat seems to concentrate on in her incessant licking of the kitten after birth. If this area is blocked off, preventing the mother from giving it stimulus, the kitten proves extremely and permanently dysfunctional. Apparently, the reticular formation fails to become fully functional if this area is missed, and the kitten then cannot process its sensory information. And the critical nature of this activation seems to be stage-specific; it must be accomplished soon after birth if it is to be done at all.

While in utero, the human infant structures certain forms of knowledge about his/her womb world, including the general sense and smell of the mother, a knowledge of her voice, perhaps her taste; and s/he is given one (at least) pattern of recognition built into his/her new brain system (otherwise rather a blank slate), the ability to recognize a face. These forms of mother recognition will help furnish his/her bondings after birth; that is, they will help to furnish points of similarity between old matrix and new, points around which s/he can assimilate the new unknown information and make an accommodation to it—if the rest of the bondings are furnished. In the new matrix, the appropriate or known voice, smell, perhaps taste, and general sensings of a primary nature must be furnished for a constant activation of those primed senses. The newborn's total sensory system must be brought into play through physical stimulus, because only by stimulation of the body does the reticular formation receive the necessary stimulus to bring *it* into full play and begin to function fully as the coordinate of body senses and mind-brain activity.

So the infant goes into an extreme stress state shortly before birth. This stimulates ACTH, which then brings about the new proteins and brain-cell connections that prepare the infant for massive and swift new learnings. The adrenal steroids prepare the body for dramatic, indeed drastic, physical changes, alerting the body and brain for the fast work to be done. And the high-stress state prepares the infant body to be highly receptive to, indeed desperate for, the particular nurturing stimuli that will reduce it. And what is that particular stimulus? It is the equivalent of the animal mother's licking. The human mother is genetically programmed to nurture the newborn's body by a continual gentle massage and stimulation, and this is what has been found in nontechnological countries.

Zaslow and Breger, in their brilliant study of infantile autism, point out the four great needs for bonding: holding, with a body molding of the infant to one's self; prolonged and steady eye contact; smiling; and soothing sounds. Breast-feeding, of course, furnishes all these at once, and body stimulus is what must be added to that vital body-molding contact.

The Ugandan mother continually massages the infant, and in carrying the infant in a sling at her breast as she resumes her daily routines, the infant is undergoing continual body stimulus. The activation of the body's sensory systems and the reticular formation is, therefore, quite rapid and complete. With a fully functional sensory system and a fully functional reticular formation to coordinate the mind-brain-body information processing and muscular responses, intelligence growth has clear sailing, for in furnishing these critical bonding needs, the mother has automatically furnished all the rest. The infant finds ample points of similarity between his/her old and new matrices. Assimilation of new information is then possible, and the brain has a fully functioning reticular mechanism for accommodation. No stage-specific portions of the biological plan are missed from a lack of preparedness, and development, swift and wonderful, unfolds according to that plan. All adrenal steroid production has completely disappeared in a short time because the infant, in being returned to and recognizing the known, relaxes. He then remains in an alert yet calm state of learning.

I will return to this bonded child later, for s/he still has more to teach us. For now, however, I need to return to the hospital-delivered infant (my five and yours, I dare say). The infant has been prepared for the greatest single act of learning or growth of intelligence ever to take place. What does the infant learn? What happens to this highly absorbent mind?

First, as Suzanne Arms has detailed so well, the entire procedure of delivery gets seriously delayed and complicated out of all bounds in hospital delivery. Drugs, particularly anesthetics, specifically slow up the synchronous movements by which the infant is expelled from the womb, and delivery gets extended to torturous lengths. Fear and anxiety build in the mother, and pain follows swift and sure. The pain calls for more medication, as does the anxiety. And what of the infant? His/her body has begun a massive outpouring of adrenal steroids preparatory to the great push and adaptation, but the movement does not come. His/her body continues its outpouring of hormones. Stress piles on stress; the expected natural cycle of stress-relaxation is not forthcoming. After hours of this, both mother and infant are exhausted.

Then there are all the medical interferences, the carelessness, and the callousness. Coupled with the conditioned reflex of fear are the operating amphitheater atmosphere, that deadly table, and being forced to lie down (or even be strapped down), which completely eliminates any last hope of muscular coordination. This is followed by drugs that incapacitate both mother and infant. (The average anesthetic passes through the placenta to the infant in forty-five seconds.³) Long before delivery (deliverance), mother and infant have been kept at a climactic point of tension, able to achieve no resolution.

What happens? Because the natural expulsion process is by now thoroughly fouled up, instrumentation is used to "assist" the mother in expelling the baby. In addition to the now commonplace practice of episiotomy (severely cutting the mother in a manner that would be considered major surgery at any other time and often causing permanent damage), forceps and suction machines are casually used to claw or suck the infant out of the mother's body, by grabbing that fantastically fragile, all too sensitive, and utterly precious head. The vast majority of the time, such instrumentation is not necessary; and only in a rare emergency could an episiotomy be justified, even with all the complications caused by the medicine man's bag of tricks. The simple truth is that he likes to use his tricks; he likes the drama and importance of his image, wielding all his mechanical toys, showing the incompetence of nature, and establishing his own superiority.

The semidrugged, overstressed, and exhausted infant is, of course, generally unable to get his/her breath, even if given ample time to do so. The many new, unused coordinates of muscles are confused and malfunctioning. His/her body is reacting only; all synchronous interactions have long since been destroyed. In addition to his/her prolonged body fear of oxygen deprivation, when s/he is finally sucked or clawed out of the mother, his/her entry is into a noisy, brilliantly lit arena of masked creatures and humming machines. (The hum of fluorescent lighting alone is an overload, much less fluorescence itself, which, as the world's greatest authority on lighting, John Ott, makes perfectly clear, is disastrous to infants.⁴) Suction devices are rammed into the mouth and nose, the eyelids peeled back to that blinding, painful light and far more painful chemicals dropped into the open eyes. S/he is held by the heels and beaten on the back or subjected to a mechanical respirator; at this critical, oxygen-short period, the umbilical cord has been cut. S/he is cleaned up a bit from the blood of the episiotomy (which will knock his/her mother out of the picture for quite some time); placed on cold, hard scales to be weighed like any other piece of meat in a factory; wrapped up (of all things, to protect him/her from those demon drafts); bundled off to a nursery crib, screaming in pain and terror if s/he is lucky; or rushed semiconscious and half dead to an incubator, far worse fate than a crib, if s/he is less lucky.

This rush is necessary because attention is focused on the cut, bleeding, injured, drugged, and depressed mother. Her comfort is the issue. Her postpartum blues will be discussed in some psychological journal, which will ask whether there really is such a syndrome. She herself, somewhere in her daze, feels that it was all so wrong. Something magnificent, earth-shaking, universal, godly, numinous, near mystical was supposed to happen and did not. She wants her baby, and all she gets are sharp commands and reprimands. Nature has done everything possible to make the newborn's venture into the unknown a success and a great learning by guaranteeing a return to the known. What the infant actually learns at birth is what the process of learning is like. S/he has moved from a soft, warm, dark, quiet, and totally nourishing place into a harsh sensory overload. S/he is physically abused, violated in a wide variety of ways, subjected to specific physical pain and insult, all of which could still be overcome, *but s/he is then isolated from his/her mother.*

It is impossible to overstate the monstrousness of this final violation of a new life. No book can ever express the full ramifications of this crime against nature. This isolation neatly cancels every possible chance for bonding, for relaxation of the birth stress, for the activation of the sensory system for its extrauterine function, and for the completion of the reticular formation for full mental-physical coordinates and learning.

The failure to return to the known matrix sets into process a chain reaction from which that organism never fully recovers. All future learning is affected. The infant body goes into shock. The absorbent mind shuts down. There will be little absorption again because there is only trauma and pain to be absorbed. The infant then surely exhibits only two states, fulfilling Spitz's expectations: "quiescence," which means semi- to full unconsciousness, and "unpleasure." If awakened from his/her survival retreat from consciousness, s/he is propelled back into a state of unresolved high stress. S/he cries him/herself to sleep again. The air of general excitement noted by Bridges surely reverts to distress. Pleasure and smiling will surely be much later in appearing, just about two and a half months later, because it will take that long for this unstimulated and isolated body to compensate if it is to survive at all. The infant's body must manage slowly to bring its own sensory system to life, get that reticular formation functioning, and come fully alive through whatever occasional physical nurturing it gets. Stage-specific processes, once missed, must be laboriously rebuilt.

During this period of shock, sensory closure, and retrenchment, there is virtually no development. How could there be? And all the other preprogrammed stage-specific developments are systematically missed, throwing the system farther behind.

Consider now the male child, whose hold on life is automatically more precarious than the female child's (see Chapter 22). In nearly all cases, the doctors circumcise the male infant on the second or third day of life. They cut off the foreskin of his penis, nearly always without anesthetic. After all, the infant—suffering excessive stress, in a state of shock, and all too often with a crippled reticular formation—seems to be a vegetable, so why not treat him as one?

Does it hurt? Of course it does. How could it help but hurt? And this is just one more of those massively negative learnings etching into that new brain-body system.

I can only dare parents, if they are going to allow this criminal act, to demand they be allowed to *watch* the performance. Just go watch, remembering that the infant registers pain just as you do. If the infant is not already in a complete state of shock before the operation, he certainly will be afterward, as parents would be if they were to observe and comprehend what is happening. Remember that the practice is a recent addition to our century's atrocities committed on children; bear in mind the growing incidence of sexual inadequacies and dysfunctions; remember that 80 percent of all silent crib deaths are male infants. Ask your doctor, though, and he will scathingly dismiss criticisms, reassure you that its perfectly all right, and make you feel rather stupid for even asking.

One of the more intriguing differences between the naturally delivered and nurtured child and the technologically delivered and abandoned child is in the matter of sleeping. Our newborns sleep massively, yet are easily awakened, in which case they cry heavily. The reason is not hard to find. Lack of physical stimulus at birth has resulted in a failure of the reticular formation's completion. Then sensory information cannot be processed properly, and sensory intake creates confusion and anxiety. The nurturings needed were also the means for reducing the high production of adrenal steroids. The combination of unrelieved birth stress and inability to assimilate and cope with sensory intake reinforce each other, they continue the flight-fight effect and adrenal overload, making the wake state intolerable.

The Ugandan child sleeps far less, is alert and awake far longer, and sleeps under a wide variety of conditions. His/her mother makes no accommodations for the infant's sleep. She carries him with her at all times and sleeps with him. During the day, he sleeps whenever the need arises, amid the hustle and bustle of his mother's daily life. Motion is the natural state for this infant, and s/he sleeps far better in motion than in stillness. Stillness, in fact, is the most alien of all states to the newborn and early infant. The Ugandan infant never leaves the known, and yet, safely ensconced with that matrix (in sling or backpack), s/he moves continually into highly stimulating new experiences. New sensory data comes pouring in with the mother right there for continual reinforcement of the basic set of conceptual patterns to which all newness can be referred. This is the ideal learning situation, an automatic stress-relaxation cycle giving continual stimulus and security.

I have mentioned that Marcelle Geber spent one year doing long-term studies of 300 of these home-delivered infants in Uganda. She used the famous Gesell tests for early intelligence, developed at Yale University's child development center. The pictures of the forty-eight-hour-old child—supported only by the forearms, bolt upright, perfect head balance and eye focus, and a marvelous intelligence shining in the face—are no more astonishing than those of the six-week-old child. At six to seven weeks, all 300 of these children crawled skillfully, could sit up by themselves, and would sit spellbound before a mirror looking at their own images for long periods. This particular ability was not to be expected in the American-European child before twenty-four weeks (six *months*) according to the Gesell tests. Between six and seven months, the Ugandan children performed the toy-box retrieval test. Geber showed the infant a toy, walked across the room, put the toy in a tall toy box; the child leaped up, ran across the room, and retrieved the toy. Besides the sensorimotor skills of walking and retrieval, the test shows that object constancy has taken place, the first great shift of logical processing in the brain, at which point an object out of sight is no longer out of mind (the characteristic of infancy and early childhood). This test, successfully completed by the Ugandan children between six and seven months of age, was not to be expected until somewhere between the fifteenth and eighteenth months in the American and European child.

Return, then, to the hospital-delivered infant, in a state of extreme stress, whisked off to that safe, germ-free nursery. Mother does need her rest, exhausted from that prolonged hard labor, dazed from surgery, badgered and drugged, plagued by a vague sense of wrongness. Hospitals do have to have their rules, of course, and even if the mother actually tries to respond to her instincts for nurturing her baby, she stands no chance at all. Scheduling is all important, you know.

One of our large daily papers ran the comments of a prominent *neonatologist* (which translates as baby doctor) discrediting the claims of Frederick LeBoyer with the casual statement: "What the newborn needs is to be kept warm and quiet, and that's what we do, we wrap them carefully and put them in a well-heated, quiet and restful place. The rest of this stuff is just nonsense."

According to rules and schedules, the time comes for a presentation to the mother. Baby is removed from the crib, jostled out of his/her sensory retreat and stress reduction, placed on a cart with the other basket cases, and trundled off for a five-minute session during which "look, but don't touch" is the rule. If feeding is part of that particular hospital's dogma, s/he may be fed, though seldom within the first few hours, and virtually never by the mother. Although the mother's milk is now known to be very much stage-specific and keyed to certain postbirth needs (of both mother and child), the hospital-delivered infant seldom gets to nurse for twenty-four hours, if then. Each of these crisply efficient awakenings propel the infant into a high-stress state all over again; again no physical nurturing takes place, and s/he is then returned to his/her crib and isolation screaming. (Everyone smiles: "Ah, a good lusty bellow in that one, obviously a fine, healthy one with a great future.")

Throughout this extremely critical transition period, then, during which the infant's brain is prepared for massive new learnings, every encounter with people is a stressful situation, with no forms of nurturing or stress-relaxation at all. At the height of this stress, the infant is isolated, which very plainly means abandoned. There, in proximity to only material things (the baby blanket), s/he must manage again to achieve some stress reduction in order to survive; the need of physical skin stimulus to facilitate this reduction finds only that baby blanket, a *nonhuman* source of stress reduction. What is the great learning? What is being built into the very fibers of that mind-brain-body system as the initial experiences of life? *Encounters with people are causes of severe, unbroken, unrelenting stress, and that stress finds its only reduction through contact with material objects.*

Consider next what the enlightened, educated, conscientious parents do when the mother and child leave the hospital. They take their infant home and set up a miniature hospital (a nursery, or at best a nursery area) to perpetuate the isolation and abandonment. After all (we have been told for generations), the little one needs his/her rest and quiet. Then there is the pervasive anxiety over germs, impelling some parents actually to wear gauze masks when near the infant for the first few weeks. Everyone tiptoes around while little junior "gets used to us," which takes, well, some two and a half months. Because silence and stillness are most alien, the infant wakes easily and screams. S/he gets colic, the symptoms of which are almost identical to those of birth stress.

S/he cries when not sleeping. No pins are sticking; no pants are wet; s/he is not cold or hungry. S/he suffers unresolved stress that builds to hyperanxiety and finally to rage, the mark of prolonged frustration. When rage appears, mother (or father) tries picking him/her up (occasionally), but the rage makes the baby hard to handle. The parent grows insecure about holding him/her, literally afraid of dropping the child. And both parents are actually a bit intimidated by this unreserved rage. They place the infant back in the crib at the height of his/her rage, so that s/he can "work off a little steam and get a good sleep."

As often as not, the parent is in a hurry, with more important things to do than pamper baby. Or if the parent is pretty hacked already, his/her own rage fires up, mixed with self-pity: "Damned if I have to put up with this." For whatever reason, the parent places the raging infant into the crib to "settle him down." That infant has been abandoned again. S/he is clearly registering and learning the meaning of abandonment, fear of which will shadow the rest of childhood and become lined with an inevitable sense of impotency.

The net result of this has been a collapsing social order, on the one hand, and a generation with an increased passion for consumer goods, on the other; and this generation can only breed more of the same. That is, the long-range effects of the materially bonded child are a breakdown of interpersonal relations and an obsessive-compulsive attachment to material objects. (A side effect, though hardly incidental, is the attempt to turn the other person into an object both because objects are capable of being manipulated and because they are not high-stress sources.)

Obsessive-compulsive attachment to objects (Linus with his security blanket, in the comic strip "Peanuts," is the tragicomic symbol of this) occurs simply because the organism learned, in its primary learnings, which take precedence over all others, that although stress comes from human encounters, relaxation or escape from stress comes from encounters with physical objects. So we have a nation—and more nations all the time as our disease spreads—in which a breakdown of interpersonal relating is coupled with obsessive-compulsive attachment to material things.

The anxiety-reduction value in any particular thing is limited, though, because it is arbitrary and unnatural and because, in the growing pressure of populations, the stress of interpersonal pressures grows continually. Anxiety is intolerable, and we will do all possible to try to alleviate it. Therefore, new objects of anxiety reduction must be had all the time. Indeed, we adults express this anxiety by propelling our children headlong into the same cycle of obsessive-compulsive acquisitions we suffer, anxious that they "get ahead in the world," which means acquire more and more things as stress reducers.

Strained as this analysis may seem, it is an accurate presentation of where we stand. Bonding is a psychological-biological state, a vital physical link that coordinates and unifies the entire biological system. Bonding seals a primary knowing that is the basis for rational thought. We are never conscious of being bonded; we are conscious only of our acute *dis*ease when we are not bonded or when we are bonded to compulsion and material things. The unbonded person (and bonding to objects is to be very much unbonded in a functional sense) will spend his/her life in a search for what bonding was designed to give: the matrix. The intelligence can never unfold as designed because it never gets beyond this primal need. All intellectual activity, no matter how developed, will be used in a search for that matrix, which will take on such guises as authenticity, making it in this world, getting somewhere.[5]

By now, I hope to have questioned your assumptions concerning intelligence, for I have found that we have no real notions of what intelligence is. I hope to convince you that human potential may be vastly beyond our current notions, for I have found an overarching framework that places both our potential and our failures into some reasonable perspective.

Before continuing with an outline of our biological plan, however, I need to clear up an issue concerning the Ugandan child. If these children are so smart, why aren't they all rich, as the old saying goes? Why aren't they all Einsteins? How come they live in those grass shacks and often starve?

All cultures that practice natural childbirth and parental bonding are (or were) cultures of *stasis*, that is, cultures based on a taboo system that prevents any novelty or change within the social body. The taboo system, or legal system, assures that no member of that culture ever makes any move that was not made by the forefathers. Every facet of these cultures works for stability. They work through stringent rules, covering every aspect of personal conduct, to prevent the unknown-unpredictable.

In Uganda, according to the strict, unbreakable custom or taboo of that culture, the mother specifically, carefully, completely, and without any forewarning, totally abandons her child when it is about four years old. She suddenly refuses even to acknowledge the child's existence. The child becomes invisible to her, as it were. The child is then sent to a distant village to be raised by relatives or is given to neighbors to raise. The psychological shock of abandonment is overwhelming to the child.[6] Severe depression develops, and many children do not survive the shock at all.

At this critical point of total vulnerability, the child is prepared for what can only be termed "bonding to the culture." The child learns the taboo system and locks into it with desperation. What s/he then learns is that to break the taboo, to act against the rules of the society, will mean banishment from that society. That would mean another abandonment, and the dread of this final and complete form of abandonment drives him/her to accept without question the strictures and qualifications the taboo system imposes. And at that point, all growth of intelligence largely stops.

Part II

The World

Chapter 8

Concept: Do You See?

Back in the 1930s, Von Senden described a new surgical operation by which cataracts could be removed and sight restored. The damaged lens was removed and special eyeglasses fitted to replace the missing lens. Eyesight was restored to many people in this way, although they experienced some tunnel vision. Attention then turned to those born with cataracts, people who had never seen anything. Should not they, too, receive the gift of vision? Alas, the case proved quite different. These congenitally blind did not see at all as expected. What they experienced was a traumatic disorientation, a confusing influx of sensory information that made no sense. They saw blotches of shifting colors that had no shape, design, or meaning. More seriously, the new sensory information coming into the system upset all the other senses: smell, taste, touch, hearing. In order to restore their orientation in the world, the patients had to close their eyes and shut out this barrage of chaotic nonsense.

Rather than a blessing, the patients felt that the operation was a curse. Many closed their eyes in a kind of survival move and refused to open them again (rather as the newborn reacts to fluorescence). Others experienced a form of hysterical blindness. Their nervous systems shut out the chaos voluntarily in an attempt to maintain homeostasis (again, as the newborn reacts to technological delivery). Some patients committed suicide (is this the true meaning of silent crib death?). Virtually none learned to see.

With congenitally blind children, the story was somewhat different. They, too, were disoriented by the new sensory information and had to close their eyes to reorient to their world. They, too, saw only shifting blotches of confused color. Childhood, however, is the period of an "unquestioned acceptance" of the given world, as Piaget put it, and some of the children were able to accept this new given. They interacted with the new sensory information through their established senses, those through which their orientation to the world had been shaped since birth. The children went up to the color blotches and interacted with them in the only ways they knew, by taste, touch, smell, hearing. They entered into an unknown-unpredictable situation with the only tools available to them, explored that unknown, and related it to their known frame of reference.

The little girl went up to the strange and meaningless blotch of color and explored it with her hands, smelled it, sensed it, and recognized it (recognized it) through her developed channels for recognition. "Oh," she exclaimed, "it's a tree, and the tree has lights in it."

This is the way any child structures a knowledge of the world. Through her interaction with the unknown-unpredictable, she opened for herself a new world of experience and possibility. She had expanded those established patterns for putting information together. Those expanded patterns then gave her a way of relating to more color blotches. Her old pattern of knowing, which identified the tree by direct sensory contact, had accommodated to the new sensory information assimilated. The tree was now more than a certain feel, smell, and general communion; the tree had lights in it.

Far more of the brain is committed to sight than to any of the other senses. Sight is the great synthesizer. It puts together all the other senses into a single, economical glance of recognition. Once she is able to see, the little girl no longer has to go through the slow, cautious, and rather perilous identification by sense, hearing, smell, and so on. Now, one swift glance places the sensory information in a context of relatedness or knowing.

Suppose I ask: What is a concept? You would probably answer: An idea. Accurate enough from an adult standpoint, but concept is not an idea in the child's mind and cannot be for several years.

Concept in the child mind is a pattern of action within the brain computer, a pattern by which sensory information is put together into a whole unit we call a *percept*. Concept is, as well, the corresponding pattern of action within the brain by which muscular response to information takes place. Any activity of the mind or body organizes and coordinates through action patterns within the brain. All those activities we call cognition, recognition, sensing, body movements, thinking, and so on are actions within the brain, momentary constructions of the brain.

Within the past few generations, and particularly within the past two decades, brain research has blossomed into an exciting and fruitful field. But a commonplace observation has been that the more we know, the less we know. The mind-brain is the most awesome and mysterious structure we know of in the universe—except perhaps that universe itself. In fact, a similarity is immediately apparent: The mind-brain is rather like a microcosm of that macrocosm. The more we study the universe, the larger and more unfathomable it becomes. The bigger our telescopes, the more rapidly it recedes from us.

Nevertheless, we surely know more and more, just as we do through brain research. Surely our unknowing about the brain grows continually, the vastness of the imponderable seems to extend even as we are gaining knowledge. Today, we are aware of how little we actually do know about the brain only because we do, in fact, know a great deal more than we used to. Our unknowing is always just as large as our knowing. Knowing and unknowing are a polarity, a yin-yang balance. It takes a certain knowledge to grasp the nature of what is not known.

We know that the brain contains about 10 billion neurons. We do not know how these neurons think or quite where thinking takes place. We know that rhythmic patterns of action and interaction between the cells go on all the time, and almost surely a similar activity occurs within individual cells themselves. We know that a single thinking cell contains upwards of 20 million huge, complex molecules, each capable of producing some 100,000 different protein complexes, all of which are almost surely involved in specific forms of information patterning.

We know that each neuron connects with other neurons through connections that are similar to telephone lines running between offices in a huge building. No line runs straight to another cell; the line connects at a point called a *synapse,* which acts as a kind of secretary taking incoming calls and directing outgoing calls. This secretary accepts only appropriate messages to relay to his/her office, and to be appropriate, the message must be similar in form to the particular pattern or form his/her office specializes in.

In an old-fashioned telephone party line, all the parties were hooked into a single wire. Each party had a ring number; perhaps yours was three rings, the Jones's next door was two, and so on. If the Smiths down the road called you, they gave three rings. Those rings sounded on all the party-line phones but were appropriate only for your house. Theoretically, only you should respond and answer (though the suspicion occasionally arose that someone sneaked that receiver off and listened in).

Among neuron telephones, a stricter propriety is maintained because a single cell may have as many as 10,000 of these direct lines branching out from it, each line in turn branching, linking that cell to anywhere from 30,000 to 600,000 other cells, each with the same paraphernalia. The number of possibilities for relaying sensory information back and forth is infinite; no number system could encompass the possibilities (particularly when we add those 20 million molecules, each capable of producing some 100,000 proteins, within each cell).

I need a model of concept structuring to clarify the way in which the infant-child structures a knowledge of the world and to show how this structure then becomes the primary process of the brain, on which all creative learning and interaction will thereafter be built.[1] Think of the brain as a large newspaper office, divided into five departments. The biggest and most important is the visual department, followed by hearing, feeling, smelling, tasting. Each department is broken down into many separate offices, each with its specific area of expertise in that particular sense medium. Each office is jammed with files and a huge array of telephone lines connecting it to other offices. Each department has specialized sensory reporters that send in messages about events out in the world. The visual reporters send messages about how the event looks; the smell reporters, about how it smells; and so on. The reporters are connected to their respective departments by long-distance telephone lines that disperse through an astonishingly streamlined office called the reticular formation. The lines between the offices pass through a secretary who screens the rhythmic character of the message to see if it is appropriate, relays the message if it is, and then informs the sender cell that the message was appropriate, which the cell relaying the message dutifully records in its files. The next time a similar message comes in, that cell will know that that particular line, among its thousands, has an appropriate rhythmic pattern for that kind of message unit.

Although each office has its specialty, just as a sports editor or an advertising editor does, each office also builds up a file system pretty much covering the activities of all the other offices through the continual cross-indexing of message relays. If really needed, any office could pinch-hit for any other. Furthermore, through the indexing and overall relay system, each office takes part in nearly all activities in one way or another. The job of the news office as a whole is to come up with an accurate composite report on the world event by putting together the various reports as they are processed by each department.

Follow a message unit coming in from a visual reporter. Hundreds of thousands of these units, or data bits, are firing in every second, but there are hundreds of millions of cells available for processing them. The message unit comes in through the central receiving office and is relayed to its appropriate department. The unit rings in its rhythmic pattern on many millions of lines ad lib, and several millions of those offices find that particular pattern appropriate to their own specialty. Office A's secretary relays the information in, meanwhile informing his/her incoming line that the message is appropriate. On receiving the information unit, the office relays the similar aspects of the message to all those offices that its files show handle similar information. The office also relays out to offices on file known to handle those particular bits of the message unit inappropriate or dissimilar to that office's specialty or precedent pattern. Finally, the office relays out on its own all-points call (ringing every line it has) that information in the message unit for which it can find no trace of precedent, no point of similarity and for which it has no record of an office that does handle such a point of information.

Office A then receives confirmations on the various appropriate targets receiving messages. Eventually, it gets back information on the more remote rundowns on offices handling the unknown, dissimilar parts of the message (those that had to be relayed out to all points). This information feeding back then gives that office a wider range of immediate relays for points of similarity and dissimilarity next time. Its own capacities have been expanded; it can take part in wider patterning of information.

When dissimilar information is rung out over the far-flung telephone network, some offices may have only a few points of similarity to that information, but these are enough to be accepted by the secretary. That office must then rerelay the remaining points of dissimilarity out on another all-points call, and this must continue until all points of information have been accounted for. This may require (in the early days) establishing new lines and using established lines in new ways.

The dissimilar items prove far more stimulating to the activities and expansion of the offices than the routine messages, but no message can be accepted and relayed unless there is some initial office with at least some points of similarity to that message. That is to say, no new experience can be accepted and interpreted unless it has at least some similarity to past experience.

Office A is continually receiving new reports directly from the sensory reporters, continually receiving confirmation and destination points of its outgoing messages to other offices, and continually receiving rings from other offices asking for similarity checks against the precedent patterns of its particlar part of the action. Office A may very well eventually get relayed back to it parts of its own messages sent out to others.

In all this welter of rhythmic activity, a pattern is worked out for some particular visual event. The pattern is the route the messages follow in being worked out into a composite interpretation by the cross-indexing of all the offices involved. These patterns between the offices get smoother and faster the more they are repeated, which means the more that experience is repeated. The secretaries develop the ability to recognize the message units handled before and do not have to check back with the office for file confirmation. Finally, confirmation of having accepted the message no longer needs to be reaffirmed. Thus, practice is the way the learning becomes engrained.

Some points of similarity are necessary in order to have some office find some appropriateness and so be able to accept the message, get it past that secretary, and get the work going on the dissimilarities. On the other hand, the department grows and becomes more sophisticated and expert in combining its overall knowledge through the influx of new information.

The department's final composite can never be found in any single office. The composite is the action of all the communications between all the offices. The composite is an instant patterning of this overall action, and the overall action becomes, through repetition, a concept or accepted editorial policy of that department. New, strange, or unprecedented reports coming in will be checked against the growing number of these patterns of precedent (concepts), which become the norm or standard of interpretation. The richer the scope of the editorial policy (the more concepts), the more complex or unprecedented reports that department can handle.

Points of dissimilarity that find only the most remote traces of similarity may require relaying back and forth many times, each relay including the particular acceptances found and the routes the information followed. This homework may run on far into the night, long after the sensory reporters have gone home to bed and the intake lines are quiet. This activity is part of a *regulatory feedback* process that goes on in the entire establishment almost all the time. Later on, in Chapters 9 and 10, we will see how this regulatory feedback works with larger and larger units of meaning, finally relaying whole concepts and groups of concepts back and forth, creating larger categories of concepts.

Finally, we come to the synthesizing, or cross-relating between departments themselves, which must be done to make an overall picture of the event. Essentially the same activity takes place, but between smelling, hearing, seeing, and so on. The department of hearing relays its composite units of information to the departments of smell, taste, sight, and feeling and receives their incoming messages in turn. Similarity-dissimilarity dispersal follows the same pattern; the references are then between the senses, and Office A, over in the sight department, will receive a cross-indexed similar-dissimilar feedback report from all the other senses and eventually know the composite of all the senses in relation to its own fixed pattern, its piece of the action.

All this takes place in milliseconds, and it takes place continually as long as consciousness is maintained. The feedback over new information may run on into the night long after consciousness has shut down. Through the continual feedback system, one office's activity might participate in virtually every conceptual activity of that particular department or even the whole plant (the entire brain). That is, no thinking cell holds a single memory item, as we used to believe. The cell is simply a possibility to be enacted by electrochemical connections with other cells in certain rhythmic relay patterns. Any cell's significance changes according to the relay pattern in which it plays a part. Office A functions rather like the typewriter key giving me letter *a*. Letter *a* can mean all sorts of different things and even sound different ways, depending on the pattern of action into which I incorporate it. In order for a neuron to think, it acts in pattern with other groups of cells, and the possibilities for such patterning are infinite.

Some of these patterns for action (concepts) are given at birth. Certain cells are preprogrammed, already wired to certain relay patterns with other cells. All it takes is a certain kind of stimulus, from a certain sensory reporter to activate this pattern. The newly hatched baby chick recognizes seeds (having a sufficient number of points of similarity to that prewired pattern) appropriate for its food. No learning is necessary, but it is still a concept in the sense that a patterning of incoming information is involved (in this case, a pattern that simultaneously acts as a coordinate of muscular responses in the body).

The newborn human has such a genetic concept for sucking when a nipple is placed in its mouth. The sensory information appropriate to this pattern is a tactile stimulus of the lips. The brain has this built-in pattern ready and waiting for just this information. The processing of these data is automatically the coordinating of a proper muscular response. We might not think of this as an intellectual act, but it so completely absorbs the baby's mind-brain system that s/he cannot attend to anything else while in this act. One concept at a time is the rule in the early days because the activation and coordinates needed are too new to allow for any division of labor.

For the newborn to recognize a face means the child is born with a concept of a face built into his/her brain cells as a pattern of action between them for handling this particular kind of stimulus. If a face is appropriate to this pattern (if there are a sufficient number of points of similarity), the infant smiles and a perception has resulted. Any face elicits a smile because any face has a sufficient number of points of similarity to be accepted and assimilated by that concept, just as the baby chick pecks indiscriminately at objects if they are approximately the right size and shape, or just as the infant will suck on your finger until s/he learns to discriminate a bit.

Where, then, is the final perception, the experience of seeing the face? Not in the eyes. The sensory reporters are there, but no single part gives the composite of the final percept. Where the perception takes place is a mystery. Obviously, the action of the brain cells and the perception of that action are for all purposes synonymous, a whole event. But perception itself does not seem to be in the gray matter, where much of the action takes place.

Evidence points toward a part of the higher brainstem as the center of awareness or the seat of consciousness, but it is probably not the point of perception. Indeed, no such point may exist at all. Just as a concept is only a pattern of action, a movement within the thinking cells, so the percept, the actual picture of the world, may be only a pattern of action or relationship between the brain as hologram and the earth as hologram. Imaginary or self-created perceptions and memory perceptions may be similar patterns of relations between individual and primary process thinking (activities to be examined in Chapters 13 and 14).

Wilder Penfield, this century's greatest brain surgeon, reported removing almost the entire hemisphere of the brain of a diseased patient without that patient's suffering loss of personal awareness, perceptions, or even memory. Furthermore, Penfield had many patients who experienced two distinct reality experiences at once. His patients had to be conscious when operated on (the brain has no feeling), and he conversed and experimented with them at great length. When Penfield electrically stimulated various areas of their brains, the patients would suddenly perceive a complete sensory replay of past events in their lives. At the same time, the patients were conscious of conversing with Penfield, of telling him of the clear sensory experiencing of some past event even as they were perceiving the operating room and the doctor. Yet, the patients were aware of each perceptual whole as distinct and knew one experience to be only memory, although it was real to the senses. Finally, the patient in each case knew of self or mind as being separate from either of the blocks of perceptual activity. This indicates, of course, that mind is distinct from the actual processes and actions of the brain (an issue to be explored in Chapters 20 and 21).

At any rate, perception (what we are aware of as that tasted, touched, felt, smelled, or heard) is the end result of a vastly complex and mysterious process. And process always means procedure, movement, action, never a specific thing. As this is true of our perceptions of the concrete world out there, so is it true of our perceptions of our own thought process, knowledge, and abilities.

Chapter 9

Cycle of Competence

Every learning unfolds in the three stages, that constitute the *cycle of competence*. First, the child goes through a period of roughing in some new ability or knowledge. Actions are clumsy and uncoordinated. Intent to do rushes ahead of ability to do. The child knows of some capacity and wishes to express that capacity immediately. The five-year-old who wished to play the piano listened to the teacher go through a "one finger, one note" explanation. The child patiently brushed this aside and explained, "You don't understand. What I want to do is go *bbbrrrmmmmmm,*" and made a corresponding magnificent sweep over the keyboard in true concert style. Unfortunately, the piano keys respond, not to that intent, but only to the ability achieved through that intent. For this reason, roughing in is occasionally a period of frustration. The new information must find corresponding patterns of similarity within the brain, be assimilated, and bring about accommodations of the points of dissimilarity, a complex set of mental-physical coordinates.

Second, a period of filling in the details follows the rough grasp achieved. The dissimilar information, requiring new neural connections and new muscular coordinations, begins to fit more smoothly. The roughed-in action begins to make sense in the repertoire of actions. Order and form begin to replace the random confusions of the earlier stage.

Third, there is a period of practice and variation, during which the new ability is repeated over and over. The myriads of synaptic threshold points become more fluid at handling the rhythmic firing of the cells in this particular coordinate.

Take as an example the probable conceptual growth based on the infant's genetic concept for recognizing a face. By using this example, I think I can show why the blind adult had such difficulty learning to see and why the child stood a better chance.

Every face coming into view activates the infant's given face concept and may elicit a smile. The neural pattern laid down in the brain responds and acts on the stimuli presented by any face to give a perception, just as any seed of the proper size and shape elicits a peck from the baby chick. The mother's face is, of course, the most frequent stimulus for the infant. The nursing infant will spend the great majority of his/her visual time staring intently at the mother's face. This constant staring roughs in a knowledge of that face and then fills in details, activating and perfecting that given concept in so doing. The infant looks off at other objects no more than about 20 percent of the time, and these are seen in relation to that face, which is the known. When s/he shifts his/her gaze back to the mother after looking at some related object or some other part of the mother, s/he is making a return to the known from the unknown. New conceptual patterns for organizing visual information are then being made in neural connections as they find or build points of similarity with the initial face pattern.

At the same time, all the infant's senses are registering the mother's presence. Nursing establishes a taste identified with her. Her smells register. The feel and texture of her skin register. (Human babies love smooth, satiny textures, just as monkey babies love rough, furry ones.) Mother's voice registers, along with her eyes looking into infant's and her smiles. All these differing sensory reports register by relating to the initial given concept for face.

Little by little, mother-face acts as a constellation for all the varied senses connected with her. Face-as-mother is roughed in, and details are filled in. Regulatory feedback, the logical ability for combining experiences into meaningful groups, slowly works toward that first constellation, the synthesis of all the sensory data through sight. Logic completes that constellation when the infant is about six months old. Under that given face concept, all the knowings about the mother are now grouped and cross-indexed. Logic achieves its first great category. Mother's face now includes all the child's structures of knowledge achieved at that point in life. She is the infant's world, extension of self, and is now known by a face that is different from all other faces. Strange faces (particularly those of strange women) may now bring, not smiles, but tears because the baby can now differentiate between faces. The number of concepts constructed by roughing in and filling in reached a critical mass, thus bringing about the constellation of all his/her knowing—not large compared with later logical achievements, but a major one at this stage.

This is the period of the *stranger syndrome.* The infant has structured a knowledge of the mother, his/her first extrauterine matrix, the goal of the biological plan for infancy. There will be more such structures of knowledge, all taking longer and involving more complex accommodations. But all future accomplishments will rest squarely on this first accomplishment and the child's continued matrix relations. The success of these matrix relations depends entirely on the permanence and stability of that matrix-mother herself.

The infant now has a safe space on which to stand. With this set of concepts, new conceptual construction will be amazingly fast. Additional points of similarity can accept experiences with greater points of dissimilarity; accommodation to these dissimilarities can give greater points of similarity. Quickly, the child's conceptual grasp leaps light-years beyond that handful of responses with which s/he was born.

Now comes the period of practice and variation. The infant must give up, so to speak, the warm security of only the mother's face. The infant faces a little birth, a small *separation from* in order to have greater relations. Here is a stranger-neighbor, whose face is a stimulus for the face concept but whose face does not fit all the other parts of the new gestalt for face that constitute the child's first structure of knowing. This new face is not also the safe space, the grounds of possibility, and the source of nurturing. All those long months of inner work have structured a knowledge that must now undergo shift and change, rather as the infant in utero is just completing his/her physical development and knowledge of that little world when s/he has to leave that knowing. This is the pattern of all growth. Once a knowledge of the matrix becomes a firm structure of knowing, that matrix must be separated from in some way, figuratively or literally, for a greater matrix, greater possibilities, and greater relations. That is, life must continually be given up for greater life, for as long as growth takes place.

So the infant must leave the known and enter into unknowns every time a stranger appears. The infant should find that interaction with the strange face does not mean loss of matrix. The strange face triggers the fear of abandonment, the greatest threat the infant and child faces and the most severe trauma that can befall him/her. The infant must find that s/he can return immediately to mother, the right face, for reassurance. Reassurance is not just some psychological sentiment; it is a replaying of, and thus reaffirmation of, the basic concepts by which the infant's structure of knowing operates. Mother's face reestablishes the known so that this unknown can find its points of similarity and be assimilated and processed. Little by little, the infant must find that the stranger (the unknown-unpredictable) does not mean abandonment or loss of matrix. S/he must find that the mother matrix is unshakable, secure, and can endure this intrusion of strangeness without dissolution.

Meanwhile, through regulatory feedback, the infant's logic of combinations is working toward the second great combinational act, one that will bring infancy to a close and usher in childhood. Through repeated experiences of distinguishing the difference between mother and stranger, with a continual safe return to the matrix, the infant begins to know that mother is permanent, that she is still there even when she is not present to the senses. S/he gains this knowing only by the mother always being there as a point of return in the encounter with strangers. Not to be there, to actually leave the child with strangers, would shatter the entire fabric being built.

Secure in the ability to return to the matrix, s/he can then separate from the mother more and more to explore, to follow his/her intent. Soon s/he is crawling and then walking. Exploring more objects with all his/her senses (tasting, touching, smelling, looking, hearing), the child's regulatory feedback receives a greater influx of newness to feed back on and structure new concepts. The conceptual system expands, giving a larger structure of knowing and corresponding physical abilities. The mind-brain's logic of combinations then moves toward its second great leap of ability. Somewhere between the age of nine and twelve months, the child's knowledge that mother is permanently there, whether immediately in sight or not, correlates to other things, shifts to a generality covering all the objects of his/her world. *Object permanency,* as Piaget calls it, takes place, a comprehensive, far-reaching logical leap in the brain. Before this time, out of sight means out of mind. After this shift, once the object is seen, s/he knows it to be permanent and there somewhere, even when it is removed from sight.

The cycle of competence found in infancy is the pattern underlying the whole period of childhood and, indeed, all the developmental stages through maturity. My example has given some indication of the superior role that vision plays in the system and of how vision is built up as a conceptual process. A final example will illustrate the move into childhood that follows the logical leap of object permanence.

Watch a twelve-month-old child exploring the vast world of his/her backyard. S/he stumbles over a stick, picks it up, looks at it long and steadily. S/he smells it, holds it to his/her chest, against the cheek. S/he chews on it a bit because taste is one of his/her best-developed identifiers. S/he does not like the gritty taste and spits. Then s/he spies the neighbor's cat crossing the walk and moves off for a new sensory venture, the stick falling forgotten.

But the stick episode is not forgotten by the child's logical feedback system. That stick event proves rich in nutrients for the mind-brain, and logic goes to work on them. That sense of the stick's smell, for instance, will be relayed back and forth through the child's patterns of precedence about smell, relating to the one primal good smell, mother. The feel of that stick will be relayed back through all tactile knowing (similar to toast, rather like cereal). But taste—ah, there is difference. S/he runs through all the categories of like and dislike, similar and dissimilar. The look of the stick will be indexed with all visual experience. The new experience's similarities with past concepts will be noted by feedback, and the dissimilarities will be accommodated by new patterning, new connections. Then the cross-indexing between the various senses will bring synthesis.

Logic will have made new connections, new patterns, which is what is meant by accommodation or adjustment. All previous concepts will have been made more flexible, with all these new connections and points of similarity established by the episode of the stick. Yet, the flexibility of any concept, its added capacity for accommodating new points of similarity, does not interfere with that concept's own original patterning. Once formed, for instance, mother-as-matrix is an inviolate pattern (unless abandonment occurs), although she becomes the source of an ever more flexible and accommodative concept.

Through the flexibility and long-range possibilities of sight, all the related concepts find a common grouping. The next time the child is walking along, s/he will recognize sticks. No longer will s/he need to pick up, feel, smell, taste each stick (though s/he may well do that for a long while) for identification. All his/her close-range sensors will be synthesized into that far more economical and rapid long-range one. In one quick glance, s/he will know what any stick probably smells, feels, tastes like. His/her logical feedback system will have grouped all the scattered bits of information from the stick experience into this single concept of stick. S/he will have structured a knowledge of stick. And all the other structures of knowledge will have been subtly enlarged and made more flexible by having to relate to this new experience.

Thus, the child's intelligence grows, which is to say, the ability to interact with the world is that much greater. His/her brain-body coordinations will have a wider and more flexible range. Each structure of knowing, each concept and constellation of concepts will be able to offer more points of similarity. This means more new experiences can be accepted and interacted with; a greater assimilation-accommodation can take place. S/he will be able to respond to more possibilities. To him/her who has, it *can* be given.

Consider the institutionalized child, isolated in a crib and given very little stimulus. His/her few given concepts find little stimulus around which to activate, practice, and expand. S/he has only his/her hands, feet, the sides of the crib, the ceiling to interact with. His/her preference for complex patterns finds little satisfaction, and above all, few faces appear for processing and interaction. Quickly, this child's logical feedback system processes every conceivable bit of experience, but the system far outstrips the intake. No nutrients come in. After a time of feeding back its limited data, all possible combinations and relations are run through and perfected. Then the system simply idles. Then it begins to atrophy. New brain-cell connections do not take place. If they do, through some trauma, no assimilable experience takes place that offers nutrients. (And, of course, these children may suffer an incomplete reticular formation from lack of body nurturing.) That for which the system is designed—the practice and perfection of logic, the ability to combine and synthesize concepts—fails to take place. The child is soon pronounced retarded, which s/he is, for retardation is usually the result of mental starvation.

Now you can see the true importance of the newborn's ability to recognize a face. This pattern gives that infant a point for the constellation of all his/her sensory impressions of his/her mother (nursing and taste, texture of skin and tactile impressions in general, smells of her milk, skin, breath, and so on). All these coalesce through logical feedback and are synthesized by sight. This means that they are all grouped together under that powerful initial pattern given: face, that base-line concept with which the infant is born. The other senses make sense in relation to that face. The face gives a point of knowing to which the other senses can relate, their varied information finding similar points of cognition.

On this cornerstone, the edifice of thinking is built. Our given concepts are remarkably few, but they are just enough. They assure us that the kinds of concepts we build will be those related to face and thus will be human concepts. Other than that, the content or nature of the concepts to be built is open. Once two or three concepts have been structured, three times that many can be structured. The possibilities quickly explode because in being born with almost no patterns at all, we learn something vastly more important than the contents of any particular concepts or all the concepts in the world. We learn to structure or create concepts, and that is the intent of the biological plan.

Now you can see why the blind child could still learn to see. Her world view or basic set of concepts had not yet firmed up, and her conceptual system was still plastic. Perhaps you can see why sight, not having been structured as the cornerstone of the conceptual system, disoriented all the senses of the patients when it came flooding in. That new sense coming in had to be cross-indexed with all the others, but it furnished no points of similarity. The relay back and forth of dissimilar information could find no possible points of similarity. This literally swamped the lines, short-circuited the entire conceptual apparatus. The experience could be neither assimilated nor accommodated, but the dominant and powerful stimuli poured right in, nevertheless. The wonder is that the little child managed to cope, that she had the muscular-mindedness to enter into that unknown and learn to see as she did.

Chapter 10

Establishing the Matrix

The mother in this chapter is a composite of real people.[1] I have met her in many different guises, in different places, in my travels lecturing on the magical child. She has not been made to feel guilty by that current accusation: "Don't you want to make something of your life?," which is heard so often in schooling when some young woman tries to follow her intent. She knows that the creation of life is the greatest of human acts and that the successful nurturing of a new life is a consummate art, greater even than being a successful accountant or advertising executive.

She conceives because she wants to create life, as her intent drives her. Her pregnancy is then first in her life and the source of her strength and calm. She knows the creative thrust of life supports her, that she is acting with the flow and has the strength of that flow. A husband may prove vital to this calm confidence, but I have met mothers who maintained their centeredness without one. I would opt strongly for the nuclear bond. I find no evidence that the ills of the culture can be laid at its doorstep, as some people claim, although the ills of the nuclear bond are almost surely culturally caused. The strength and support of a husband or mate is almost essential for an anxiety-free pregnancy and mothering. The role of the father as a transitional figure from mother to world, particularly after the child's second year, cannot be overstressed. I am leaving fathers out here simply because the strength and response of the mother is the issue. His strength must feed into hers and through hers to the new life. That is the way nature has designed the process.

This mother is responsible, able to respond. She responds to the needs of her body with the same respect and care she will show for her infant in and out of the womb. She responds by making her own preparations for delivery, birth, and bonding. During the last months of pregnancy, she works specifically for bonding with her unborn child. She may have a simple tune she hums to her infant over and over. She will sing or hum this same tune during delivery and birth as one of her many bonding cues. She talks aloud to him/her continually because she knows that the infant hears and responds physically with synchronous body movements.

She keeps communion with the child, thinking positive and creative thoughts about him/her. They are already friends. She attends to her child, becomes aware of different movements and responses. She is, from the first signs within her, learning about her child, learning to take her cues from it and respond accordingly.[2]

Knowing anxiety to be the great crippler of intelligence, she works purposely for a calm repose. She begins each day in quiet meditation, establishing her union with the flow of life and with her child. She closes each day in the same way and makes her time in between a living meditation, a communion and rapport, a quieting of the mind to tune in on the inner signals. She reduces all the fragmenting intentions of life to the single intent of her act of creation.

She does not indulge in doubt. She chooses what she will entertain in her mind, and she chooses confidence, which means moving with faith. She knows the contents of her mind are matters of her own choice, that anxiety contents stir adrenal steroids that are passed on to her child.

She may elect to deliver her child herself, with or without help. She does not break the even tenor of her days but continues in her life routines. She avoids the risk of serious startle or stress, knowing the adrenal flood would transfer to her infant. She prepares a proper delivery and birthing place: private, quiet, dimly lit, with no possibility of unwanted intrusion or noise. The necessities for tidying up are laid out, and a warm bath may be readied. The preliminary signals are noticed with rising anticipation and excitement, but without alarm. Relieved of the trauma of having to rush off to a hospital, she continues her routines until the final moment.

If she has help (the midwife, perhaps a doctor, and the father), they are there only for the physical delivery itself. They maintain quiet and calm, giving strength and support. Onlookers and friends distract, break the flow, set up expectancies discordant with the flow of the event. Her intent and intentions must merge into a single point of total absorption. She uses the birthing position adopted throughout the ages, squatting on her haunches or perhaps on her knees. This aligns her with the earth, with gravity, puts all her muscles into the most advantageous positions for the work at hand. She flows with the process, a balance of stresses and relaxations.

She knows what to do by heeding the 3-billion-year biological coding built into her genes. Her knowing is not articulated, thought-out, coherent, or verbal. She is just a coordinate of smooth actions. Her thought is her body action, and in this she is like a child. She is gripped by that same intensity found in deep play (skiing a dangerous slope, scaling a cliff face, fast tennis): the total attentiveness and single-mindedness of confrontation, an ultimate encounter. Every move, act, signal heeded is an unbroken flow of controlled abandon. By being responsible, she is in her power, a joyful response to a body-knowing that "breathes" her and does the proper thing at the proper time.

If there is pain, it is the white intensity of pain without the hurt of it, and that intensity is power. She knows the intensity of this absolute exertion from the many acts in her life building her current muscular-mindedness, her ability to enter into the unknown and unpredictable. This heady joy of personal power, this grand, illuminated understanding is hers through her complete response, her total *yes* unmarred by fear or doubt: the knowing that she *is* the flow, the life process, the nexus of power, the meeting point of creation, the matrix from whom all things flow.

Her relaxed alertness keeps her supple as needed, and the journey is quickly accomplished. After all, the distance is remarkably short. The head appears. Immediately, the newborn takes a sharp breath and gives a startled cry. Air in his/her new, unused lungs is unpleasant and hurts. S/he may not breathe again for half a minute or longer. Meanwhile, the mother may slip her fingers beneath the infant's armpits and help it out, the tiny body simple to remove after that enormous head. Avoiding any sudden or strenuous movement, she takes the infant, leans slowly back, and gently places him/her, belly down, to her breast, his/her body molding to the very contours of the belly s/he has just left. S/he has left that known matrix and entered into a new one, and yet here s/he returns to the known, though in a new form.

She does not touch the infant's head except to support it as needed in lifting it to her stomach. Then, with her hands cradling him/her as her womb did, she leaves the child alone. She is humming her tune now, and the child takes another cautious breath as his/her intent prompts. S/he has no need for hurry because s/he is still drawing blood and oxygen from the mother. The cord is, of course, intact. The newborn's heart has not yet made its full transition of sending blood to the lungs, a transition that will take several minutes and for which the billions of years of preparation have not failed to equip the child. With the double source of oxygen available, the transition is calm and gentle.

Safely on her belly, the baby begins to relax. S/he has picked up the mother's familiar heartbeat and hears her familiar hum. Points of similarity are beginning to emerge. S/he breathes cautiously and tentatively as prompted, crying a bit at the newness, and breathes more regularly, each breath easier. Within a few minutes, breathing is steady and regular, as the mucus in the tubes clears. His/her contact with the mother's nipples triggers the afterbirth into play; the contractions of the discharge of the placenta aid in sending the final reserves of blood and oxygen to the infant.

At this point, any others in the room leave. This first hour after birth is the most critical time in human life.[3] For now the bond is established in strange, mysterious, and unfathomable ways. Anyone else around literally gets caught in the magnetic fields of attraction weaving back and forth. A great love affair is being born, a love affair that is sensuous, sexual, spiritual, mental, quietly ecstatic. As Marshall Klaus puts it, "they must learn to make love with each other." The self has divided and reunites with the self. The hologram part starts immediately moving into and reflecting the whole. Only in the great second bonding, many years hence, will life again enter into this same ecstacy.

The baby's arm moves; s/he extends a hand, exploring, touching, searching for familiar barrier cushions. The other arm follows; the legs extend. The mother gives her infant her hands to push against, establishing a temporary boundary to this now boundless world, lest this new freedom be overwhelming. Slowly, his/her entire body begins movement, and the mother begins a slow, gentle massage that will continue off and on for weeks. Beginning with the infant's back, she caresses with her hands in slow, rhythmic, and very light movements, stimulating his/her entire body, working the fatty vernix caseosa into the skin. This continual stimulation activates many physical processes (digestive, eliminative, sensory, and those of the reticular formation that had to await delivery to be enacted). Delivery stress has flooded him/her with arousal hormones, and massive new neuronal connections have been made within the brain, preparatory for this great learning s/he is now embarked on. Now her nurturing quiets the stress, reduces the hormone production, and furnishes the child with the basis of a learning that builds into the very fiber of body and mind. S/he is learning that learning, the movement from the known into the unknown, can be joyful.

The mother has paid no attention to the placenta discharging, having too many other cues to respond to. She cuts the cord at leisure. No suturing or tying is needed because the blood vessels have long since completed their assignment and shut down.

She may elect to place the baby in the little tub of warm water she has prepared.[4] Naturally, she does not use soap; s/he could not possibly be dirty, and all the vernix needs to be absorbed eventually. The bath is to furnish an environment similar to the one s/he has left. She makes her decisions according to cues from the infant. She does everything possible to furnish an environment with points of similarity to his/her former matrix, to complete a cycle of stress-relaxation by making newness compatible with the known s/he has left. Thus, the new system will not suffer sensory overload and withdraw into one of the minor forms of shock. There are too many stage-specific processes opening at this point that prove vital to future learning. She knows that s/he is involved in the most strenuous act of intelligence s/he will experience in life.

S/he floats in the warm bath, assisted by the gentlest support from his/her mother. Here s/he truly awakes. The mind-brain system begins a rapid transition to the new environment because a fluid environment is familiar. Now s/he opens his/her eyes wide and full and keeps them open in the gentle light, looking, looking. Those eyes register the inner-intent question that will drive the child unceasingly forward during the next seven years: Where am I? What place is this? Out of this driving quest will come his/her structuring of knowledge of the earth and life.

The bath is leisurely because s/he is in his/her element now and all senses waken. She may introduce the child to a bit more light. If daylight has broken, she raises the shade a bit. S/he will turn and stare at daylight for long periods. She does not use electric light, which creates sensory overload. The baby's hands are open, relaxed, exploring. S/he looks at them, chews on the fingers a bit. S/he is in continual movement, with mother's hands gently massaging him/her in the water.

The mother dries her baby and returns it to her body when s/he shows signs of distress. She may nurse the child, the nursing furthering the tightening up of her abdominal muscles.[5] This early milk may contain hormones that further the act of bonding and contribute to the final dispersement of birth stress. She molds the infant to her, maintains eye contact, smiles, hums, and talks. If it is dawn, she may open a window to let the child hear birdsong. Nestled together, they warm each other as designed. She may play a bit of quiet music to introduce sounds other than her heartbeat and her voice. Because the mother introduces the infant to the elements of the world gently and one at a time, his/her senses are brought into play, easily and gently, as all aspects of this new life have been. That reticular formation in the child's midbrain becomes fully activated, and all the growth processes that are stage-specific to birth begin to function on schedule.

Within hours, the newborn is smiling. Initial excitement has converted to joy. S/he knows where s/he stands: in the safe place, the matrix. S/he is bonding. At no point has this new sensory system been overloaded with excess stimuli or stimuli beyond his/her ability to assimilate and accommodate. All has been orderly, calm, and quiet, yet with a constant stimulus from the matrix source. S/he has undergone the greatest learning of life, moved from a known to the unknown of the most extreme sort, and found this movement to be a source of strength or comfort. S/he has been given the great strength of the new matrix. S/he has found nurturing; his/her body needs have been met. S/he has experienced the relaxation of birth stress. S/he is learning that in giving up life as known, one enters into greater life. This is the source of muscular-mindedness, the strength of intellect to accept the great gift given.

Within hours, the mother resumes the routines of her ordinary life. The baby is never separated from her. She knows that abandonment is the most severe trauma that can befall a child, that the threat of abandonment is the severest anxiety that a child can undergo, that anxiety quickly cripples the growth of intelligence. She takes no chance of even the slightest break in this tenuous new bond; she avoids any event that might even bring the automatic assurance of it into question. She knows that the breaking of the bond or even ruptures in it form as permanent body-knowing.

She sleeps with her infant. There will be no silent crib death here, for there is no crib. There will be no sudden unheeded drop in blood sugar, for nourishment is always there for him/her. S/he will feed from fifty to sixty times a day. The mother carries her infant with her throughout the day in a sling in front, where eye contact can be maintained and body molding kept intact, and where s/he is kept at just the right temperature.[6] Later, she may use a back carrier, papoose style. S/he sleeps at any time, as needed, wherever they are, whatever they are doing. The mother makes no accommodation to the infant's sleeping. S/he is far more used to movement and some noise than to stillness and total quiet and sleeps easily and well as the mother goes about her work.

Yet, the baby sleeps surprisingly little. Life in this new world is simply too exciting; there is too much going on. Not only is s/he never separated from his/her matrix, but also s/he is continually moving into unknown situations while safely ensconced in the known. This is the ideal learning situation, which the biological plan has designed for all intellectual growth throughout life. S/he is finding that learning is not movement *from* the known into the unknown, but movement *of* the known into the unknown. S/he is finding that his/her matrix is movable.

The daily strangeness s/he encounters all relates to the matrix. The world they move through is an extension of the mother and so of the child. The strangeness is by and large the same, and familiarity is soon established. The known is expanding to include the environment of the matrix (the family and house), at least in roughed-in conceptual form.

The sensory stimuli for vision and hearing are continuous and uncontrived. When sensory overload comes about, as it does continually, s/he simply drops off to sleep. This shuts out further sensory stimuli and allows regulatory feedback to catch up in its computing of new information.

S/he explores the mother constantly. While nursing, the infant spends most of his/her visual time on her face, in direct eye contact. S/he cannot focus his/her eyes and suck at the same time; any sensorimotor act is totally engrossing at this early stage. S/he looks away part of the time and then swings back to the known, reinforcing the basic patterns for sensory organization. The vast importance of being given the mother's face from the beginning is that the conceptual system the child builds rests on this first point of knowing. A fear of abandonment in the older infant and child is not a simple fear of losing his/her source of nourishment, or object attachment, as psychoanalytic people call it. Far more important than the problem of nourishment or even ease of body stress, fear of abandonment is based on fear of a threat of a collapse into chaos, a loss of the means for concept structuring. Mother is his/her conceptual channel for interacting and responding to the world as intent prompts him/her to do. Mother represents the building block, the cornerstone of meaning, the pattern around which the child's mind-brain structures its whole body of knowledge. The infant-child must have a constant reinforcement of this basic structure if new experience is to be continually accommodated.

The great fortune of the magical infant is that his/her base line of conceptual patterns receives continual reinforcement at the very time s/he receives a continual stream of new stimuli. At the same time, his/her body is receiving continual stimulus from the movements of the mother, providing a continual enhancement of the nervous system. His/her system receives the right balance of stimuli to maintain alertness, the accompanying hormones producing a proper growth of proteins in the brain, providing ample growth of new neuronal connections, stimulating this growth in proper synchrony with the input of new information.

In their bonding interactions, the infant establishes rapport with the mother as she does with him/her. S/he responds to cues from the mother as readily as she responds to him/her. S/he is biologically geared to take cues from the mother from the beginning, as an aid in world-view structuring. Quickly, infant scheduling coordinates with hers; s/he atunes to the mother's sleep patterns (daytime grows too interesting to miss). Just as two women in the same household often fall into the same menstrual cycle, so the infant begins to reflect the mother's general life rhythms. She has few sleepless nights with her baby. By never separating in these critical early days, the mother is surprisingly free of the child in comparison with the average anxiety-ridden parents during those first ten to twelve weeks of adjustment.

She watches her child and responds to his/her movements. Remember that the infant's brain has been prepared for many new learnings at this period, far more than we may know or respond to. Just as his/her so-called random movements will immediately synchronize with speech used around him/her, s/he has many other preprogrammed movements. If the significance of these cues is missed, they go unnurtured.

Within the first day of the baby's life, the mother may elect to start arbitrarily sitting him/her up, helping him/her to achieve head balance. Soon she is holding the baby by the forearms, easing him/her into a sitting position as s/he achieves the needed head balance. She repeats the performance many times during those times of the infant's daily cycle in which the peculiar alertness characteristic of learning is apparent. (Klaus has charted this rhythmic cycle of the infant's day.) At each repetition, those bodily movements themselves bring about a corresponding rhythmic pattern of action in the infant's computer brain. Although these body movements are part of the overall intent, it would take the infant a long time to discover them and a great deal of laborious effort to achieve control over them if s/he was left to his/her own devices. Intent must be given content. Although s/he is preprogrammed to respond to speech, the infant might be slow to speak if s/he is given no models.

In this highly absorbent learning period, the infant's brain automatically patterns body movements, even when those movements are induced from without. During this period, the brain is rather like one of those etch-a-sketch devices: Make this movement down here, and the pattern etches in up here.

Once those patterns form, each repetition strengthens them. This soon leads to volitional control; the infant can finally begin to initiate and execute such movements. This is sensorimotor learning and helps explain the precocity of the Ugandan infant.

The mother stimulates her infant in many ways. Taking her cues from the baby's subtle movements and indications of being in a learning period, she amplifies his/her movements and then repeats them. When the infant starts to grasp for an object, she makes sure that movement is successful and encourages repetitions. Because the mother also senses his/her general state and responds to needs even as they arise, the infant learns that when s/he gestures toward the matrix, that matrix gestures back, greatly expanding his/her personal capacities. Muscular-mindedness grows this way. The full significance of this will unfold when the child is around age seven, with the development of operational thinking. Nothing leads to personal power like successful moves of personal power. Success breeds success.

In no way is the mother beguiled by such nonsense as the notion that things must not be too easy for her infant, lest s/he think the world is a bed of roses. She knows that frustration does not build concepts in the brain. Concepts for interaction build through successful assimilations (the ability to accept and digest new experience), and successful accommodations (new patterning to handle dissimilarities and make new muscular coordinations of response). Success in stress-relaxation is success in adapting unknowns to the known. The mother knows that the infant is prompted from within by an enormous drive that goes ahead of ability. And she knows that there are frustrations aplenty in that.

Success gives the infant-child the ability to accept the stress of intent preceding ability; it gives him/her the patience to persevere in the face of initial discouragement. In the future, when reach exceeds grasp, s/he will persist in his/her attempts exactly to the extent that s/he has succeeded previously. Initial learnings determine the pattern and attitudes by which further learning unfolds. If failure is built in from the beginning, frustration overrides success, stress does not resolve to relaxation, the entire process of sensorimotor development slows.

The mother knows that throughout infancy and early childhood, the child is *egocentric*, that s/he does not distinguish between subject and object, between in here and out there. S/he is both the center of the universe and that universe. All radiates out from the child. The world out there is but an extension of self, and the ability to affect that world is equivalent to control and power. The mother is part of this egocentrism. She is in a real sense the infant's larger self, his/her world, and the content of that world. When the mother takes her cues from the child and responds to his/her movements, assisting in sensorimotor awakening, the world is meeting him/her halfway. A true interaction is then taking place, a dynamic exchange of energy between world and that world's offspring, as found in every living plant and animal.

By relating the items and events of the world to the mother-matrix, the infant's conceptual framework builds very rapidly, for the secure intellect can absorb information and experience at a truly incredible rate. On the other hand, anxiety, or lack of bonding, forces the intelligence to try to secure for itself some safe place while attending to the drive to move outward. As in the case of sucking the nipple and focusing the eyes, the system cannot attend to two drives simultaneously, and the drive of anxiety (turning back to look for the matrix) overshadows all others in the beginning and throughout life.

Quickly, the biological plan provides new tools for the child's interactions with the world. S/he learns to grasp for and seize objects, and this opens a full-dimensional interaction with the materials of the family world. Before this, s/he had to depend considerably upon the long-range senses of sight and sound for interacting with those objects related to, near, and around the mother. This, along with the tactile explorations of the mother, provided plenty of information for the new conceptual system. But now, a full-dimensional sensory interaction is possible. When called for, the need is provided for because the child's conceptual system now has a sufficient number of basic patterns around which additional constellations of sensory patterns can be grouped and related.

Because grasping and holding provide possibilities for tasting, feeling, and smelling, as well as looking, his/her conceptual frameworks cross-index and form constellations at a faster and richer level. Once sitting up is accomplished, crawling develops, and that expands the world of graspable objects just as the infant is ready for this expansion. S/he can now interact with the microcosm of his/her household, moving from object to object, exploring, building full-dimensional structures of knowledge.

For some time, the infant has been making those random speech sounds that prepare for articulate word imitation. "Mamma," for instance, is a universally produced lalling sound, and it is picked up by all parents and repeated back to baby. In this kind of imitation, the infant's own sounds elicit a response from the world and lead directly to his/her imitating the sounds s/he hears, just as his/her extensive body movements have prepared him/her to do. Mother talks to the child continually, in ordinary, everyday tones and manner. She knows she cannot teach the child to speak. Intent drives him/her toward that, and by the end of the first year, s/he may have learned considerable language. (Or s/he may not. Speech is not so critical in its stage-specificity. Einstein, for instance, did not speak until three years of age.)

Standing follows crawling and is followed by the fail-safe practice of falling by sitting that precedes walking. Between the ages of eight and ten months, the infant may begin walking. Once the enormous coordination of actions involved in walking are comparatively smooth, the one-act-at-a-time system can turn its attention to talking. (Some children talk before walking, however, so in this development there is no hard rule.) In all these learnings, mother meets child halfway, assisting him/her, assuring success, giving strength. The child's autonomy unfolds rapidly, making the mother's assistance less and less necessary.

The stranger syndrome indicates a qualitative shift of logic around the age of six months, as noted earlier. (And in a highly mobile, crowded metropolitan environment, where new faces are everyday affairs, this syndrome might not appear, although mother-face constancy, the preliminary to object constancy, still takes place.) As the child learns to accept strange faces and finds that his/her matrix is always there, his/her logic of combinations correlates and groups object experiences accordingly. This leads to object permanence or constancy, his second shift of logic.

From the moment s/he could crawl, the infant would spot an object, zero in on it, and move toward that object with single-minded intent, ignoring everything else. If mother did not want the child interacting with some object, all she had to do was move that object out of sight. She simply pushed father's watch behind a book, and baby immediately shifted focus to another object, zeroed in on that, and so on. One day, without preamble, somewhere between eight and twelve months, this effect no longer takes place. Mother has moved the Dresden figurine behind the flowerpot and off s/he goes, around the pot, looking for that out-of-bounds figurine. The object out of sight is no longer out of mind. Now the child knows that the object is still there somewhere, although it is no longer present to his senses. So mother has to resort to other devices with inappropriate objects. Infancy has come to an end.

A major, fundamental shift of logic has taken place. The child's ability to process information from the world has undergone one of its dramatic changes. In addition to the one-for-one correspondence with the world, his/her brain computer can now retain knowledge of an object's presence in the world even when there is no sensory stimulus from that object. Exactly how such symbolic knowing takes place is not clear, but it takes place suddenly and changes all information processing. The logic of constancy is probably an ability to hold a visual pattern as a possibility of construction, simply awaiting the reappearance of the proper stimulus, much as the infant knew that mother was the proper stimulus for face.

Every operation within the brain is now different. Logic has achieved its first flexibility, and intelligence truly opens. Knowledge of the matrix has been structured. The child now has a safe place to stand. His/her attention can now shift away from a sole compelling interest in the mother because she is now axiomatic, the basis of thought—and so not thought about, just assumed. His/her intellectual energies no longer need to center there. From now on, mother *is* the center from which s/he will move out and away, although continually returning to her for reinforcement of conceptual sets and renewal of personal power.

Now his/her intent moves into the living world, into every nook and cranny of the household and into the world outside. The question "Where am I?" moves to encompass the matrix of all matrices, the earth itself. Childhood begins as s/he moves to interact with this living earth and structure a knowledge of it, just as s/he has structured a knowledge of the mother, for the living earth must eventually become the matrix if the biological plan is to proceed.

Chapter 11

World As It Is

Nature programs the child to do two things from ages one to seven: structure a knowledge of the world exactly as it is, on the one hand, and play with that world in ways that it is not, on the other. In this chapter, I will discuss the work of structuring, play is discussed in Chapter 15.

Structuring a knowledge of the world takes at least six years because the world is filled with many things and its processes and principles are strict. The child is programmed to interact with the actual world: a place of rocks, trees, grass, bugs, sun, moon, wind, clouds, rain, snow, and a million things; a world that runs on principles, where cause and effect balance, where "fall down, go boom" means skinned knees, where fire burns and hot means don't touch.

The world is a very practical place, and nature provides the child with a very practical intelligence: his/her ability to interact through the five senses and body movements. Nothing more is needed. Concepts are very much the issue of intelligence in childhood (and throughout our lives). New patterns for sensory organization and bodily action form in the child's brain only as s/he interacts with the world through the body. Throughout childhood, a full-dimensional and accurate concept is an internalization of an external act.

All children tend to stare vacantly for long periods. Burton White finds that the brightest children are those who are allowed to stare without interruption. Staring may rough-in visual concepts as empty categories in the brain to be filled in later by full sensory interaction. Many of the patterns in the brain cannot be more than one- or two-dimensional concepts, for example, as patterns for visual organization to which other senses do not apply. However, an accurate knowledge of the world depends on full-dimensional concepts structured from a cross-indexing of all the senses appropriate. One- and two-dimensional concepts cannot be interrelated by regulatory feedback to form the critical mass necessary to shift matrix from mother to earth.

It took many months for the infant to form enough full sensory patterns relating to mother to give the critical mass and logical shift of face constancy and the formation of mother as matrix. It took a certain critical mass of tangible sensorimotor interactions with real things for the shift of logic to object constancy, ushering in childhood. The necessary critical mass of concepts about that world exactly as it is must accumulate for regulatory feedback to organize and synthesize. Around age seven, a dramatic shift of brain growth and logic will occur. The child's matrix will (or should) shift from the mother to the earth. S/he will then have the living earth as the place of power, the safe space, and the source of possibility. The child will be bonded to that earth. These bondings will grow until his/her ability to interact opens to breathtaking dimensions.

For most of us this bonding to the world, or matrix shift, is blocked by anxiety in much the same way that bonding to the mother is crippled or warped. Earlier I showed how bonding at birth was crippled, and later I will show how bonding to the earth is crippled. For now, though, I need to present evidence for a bonded child bonding to his/her earth at the stage-specific time.

This transition from mother to world ideally involves both parents, although the father is never a substitute matrix (unless the mother dies). Nature has designed it so that mother is matrix. Father is vital as the bridge from mother to the world somewhere in that second year of life and to the larger world of society around age seven. Father draws the child out from a symbiotic kind of relation with the matrix into ever larger matrices. But each matrix shift encompasses the former. Alienation or isolation from a matrix is destructive. Father is the bridge from symbiotic to creative relationships, the ability to leave freely in order to interact creatively with the matrix. This drawing out is like the sun's drawing of moisture from the earth in order to send that moisture back in a life-giving rain. Father and mother are rather the stress-relaxation poles for the child: The father is the pull into the unknown; the mother is the known, the touchstone. In balance and harmony, they provide the perfect ground for growth.

Therefore, I will refer from now on to parent or parents, rather than to just mother. The parents work for the child's intellectual strength, which rests on the richness and fullness of his/her concepts, which, in turn, build through his/her interactions with the world. The parents know that the biological plan leads toward the earth becoming the child's matrix, with a creative logic unfolding by which the child's physical survival in that world can be secured.

One issue that the parents keep uppermost in mind because it is easy to forget is that the child's logic and their logic are different ways for processing information. They do not confuse their reality experience with the child's reality experience. Their rule is never to describe any aspect of the world to their child by word or implication. Their education of him/her is into the world as it is, free of adult values placed on it.

The child is driven to acquire a completely nonspecific or unconditional knowledge of the world. S/he is designed and equipped to acquire information and experience free of value, meaning, purpose, or utility. Adults tend to value all experience and knowledge according to cultural ideas about utility or worth. An intelligence cued to look for the worth or utility of information or experience immediately closes or screens possibility, looking for what can be utilized. An open intelligence and a flexible logic cannot be built this way, although a facile cleverness that can pass for brilliance in our culture's anxiety-ridden body of knowledge might then develop.

The largest source of misunderstanding between parent and child may be in the child's lack of concern over value and utility. Because adult life is based on such concerns, the child's unconcern is a source of anxiety for the parents. But only if the child is allowed to experience the world without concern for its value or utility can s/he build a knowledge of that world as it is—because the world has no values. Only through an open and unvalued knowledge of the world can a practical and realistic value and utility form when the biological plan needs such evaluation. This need does not (should not) arise at all until the shift of matrix from mother to earth around age seven, a shift that is, ironically, partly dependent upon the child's structuring of his world view free of arbitrary or premature value or judgment.

The parents know that their child's brain system structures concepts from his/her direct sensory interaction with material things and actual processes. They let the child alone unless s/he indicates need. They let him/her roam the house freely because its contents are a major source of early world knowledge. They play with their child as they find time and as s/he indicates a need. They talk to the child continually in fully adult style. S/he loves their household conversations and listens intently long before s/he has a vocabulary for grasping their meaning. This fascination for conversation is a kind of aural staring.

Actual communication with the child is another matter. The parents' rule for communications of instruction, demands for compliance, or response to queries is: Unless s/he can touch, taste, feel, smell, hear what they refer to, no communication takes place. Abstract communication (not referring to the immediate context), particularly if the child is expected to respond or obey, creates the same kind of sensory disorientation in his/her brain that sight created in the congenitally blind.

The parents know that the child's survival is their concern, that the reason for the exceptionally long dependency of the human child is precisely that s/he might not have to be responsible for his/her own survival throughout the formative years. Only by being kept completely free of survival as an issue can the child construct a value-free knowledge of the world. And only by remaining valueless can knowledge remain open and logic flexible, openness and flexibility infinitely beyond that needed for survival in its ordinary evolutionary sense but that will lead eventually to an efficient and practical way of survival itself.

The child is designed to structure knowledge only to develop the tools of intelligence and logic, the ability to interact. What s/he interacts with is never so important as the knowledge of, or ability for, interaction s/he gains from that encounter. The biological plan is a drive for knowledge as ability, not knowledge as information. Information is of value only as it enhances the ability to interact. Once this ability develops, the information through which the development took place is incidental, and no longer of value.

Acquisition of content is an obsession with adults who have no matrix. When the resulting value system is forced on the child and acquisition of content becomes the child's thrust, intent collapses into intention. The intellectual system then closes in on the specific content valued, whether that content be material goods, idea systems, or self-images. This closure immediately cripples the ability to interact. The growth of intelligence bogs down, as intelligence tries to create a static situation centered on the valued content. This is impossible. In a universe in which everything must move and flow in order to exist, only ability to interact with that flow is of value. This is what the child intuitively knows and strives to maintain.

If the child's security with parents is unquestioned, then his/her concern over survival will never become an issue. The child is designed to enter into experience freely, without prejudgment, and evaluate that experience after it takes place. Concern over survival, safety, or well-being immediately forces an evaluation of experience before that experience can take place. Such concern immediately fires into effect some form of flight-fight arousal, which then screens all present and potential for its flight-fight value (its potential for the child's harm or well-being). This ties intelligence into a decision based on the value of the experience. There is then no unquestioned acceptancy of the given, which is the hallmark of the whole child. Anxiety over survival causes a screening of information through the question: Am I safe? The bonded child does not formulate this question. The bonded child asks only, Where am I?, and moves to interact accordingly.

Once anxiety over safety becomes a child's orientation, s/he will use his/her long-range senses (sight and sound) as buffers between self and experience. S/he will try to predetermine the probable value and outcome of the experience in an effort to keep distance between him/herself and possible harm. S/he will use intelligence to try to determine a direction offering escape from anxiety. Overdependence on long-range senses means, in turn, a failure to interact with the world on a full sensory level. A concrete knowledge of the world as it actually is, with ironclad principles of cause and effect, is then never fully grasped. A knowledge of the matrix does not become fully formed, just as the infant in utero flooded continually by adrenal steroids from an anxiety-ridden mother fails to develop fully. A shift of matrix at age seven becomes highly problematic because that structure of knowledge is insufficient. Matrix shifts take place according to genetic timing, not preparation. When the preparation is incomplete, the new matrix is incomplete, the shift is still away from the old, and the unfortunate child is left stranded.

Anxiety is always the enemy of intelligence and always blocks the biological plan. The minute anxiety arises, intelligence closes to a search for anything that will relieve the anxiety. This might lead to the street-smart mentality or to precocity along narrow culturally approved lines, but the biological plan will have been aborted.

Most parents force a concern for value on their children prematurely. Adult value, almost without exception, has its basis in a concern over personal survival, well-being, or avoidance of anxiety. So the parents of the magical child assume his/her survival for him/her and do everything possible to keep any notions of survival or anxiety over survival from forming in his/her mind. Because s/he is biologically geared to take his/her cues from them and to pattern his/her world structuring after them, they must practice their faith in the biological plan and keep their relations with him/her free of anxiety. A child bonded to anxiety cannot help becoming anxious.

Value in this adult anxiety sense and like-dislike in the child sense are not at all the same things. The child will certainly like or dislike almost every experience s/he undergoes. But s/he likes or dislikes only after the fact of having had the experience, not before. When s/he randomly picks up a stick and chews on it for taste identification, s/he spits because s/he does not like the taste. "This item is not good for eating" enters his/her feedback concerning the concept of stick. Such like-dislike evaluations arising from experience are not negative experiences. The child, initially at least, has no logical process for going around looking at objects and saying, ahead of time, "I don't think I like that because I'll bet it doesn't taste good." His/her roughed-in knowledge of the world could never form that way. S/he is neutral toward experience and simply driven to it.

His/her evaluations are a result of experience, and s/he does not correlate judgments. That is, s/he does not stop putting objects in the mouth to taste-identify them because the stick did not taste good. Not even sticks, necessarily. The child is impelled throughout this roughing-in stage to interact with every object with every sense available or appropriate. We lament this ("Why can't s/he learn not to put things in his/her mouth?") not realizing the vast negative learning in violation of his/her genetic drive that would demand. His/her drive impels him/her to enter into each experience anew, without qualification or condition, in order to construct a concept of that experience exactly as it is.

The child's openness concerning value depends on being allowed to form like-dislike opinions about experience. That is, s/he must be allowed to decide for him/herself whether an experience is good or bad. S/he must have the *option* of deciding, and his/her decisions must be honored. Otherwise, closure of intelligence will take place.

The parents make available to their child every possible opportunity for exploring the world, both the human world of artifacts and the natural world. To the extent that the child's world is open and available to his/her driving intent, to that extent s/he will accept boundaries and restrictions. Remember that the child is biologically geared to take his/her cues from the parents. Obviously, there must be boundaries, the child needs them. Boundaries give his/her world structure. Although there should be no restraints on the child's exploration of his/her physical world in a natural state, if you have railroad tracks running through your backyard, that third rail must obviously be out of bounds. But it takes just such a stringent possibility to justify curbing the child's exploration of the world. Surely there must be boundaries concerning property, persons, the rights of family members, and so on, but these are few unless arbitrarily fussed over, and the child will take his/her cues surprisingly well if the lines of relationship are clearly drawn.

The parents do not subject the child to situations in which arbitrary boundaries block his/her biological thrust toward exploration. They do not take the eighteen-month-old into a public restaurant for a few leisurely hours, because they know that s/he cannot interact with such a world for long. They know that s/he has no logical machinery for grasping the subtleties of a blocked situation, that s/he has only intent driving him/her. They know that situations blocking intent produce anxiety, so they do not tempt him/her with situations offering only frustration. They are responsible for their child, and they recognize that his/her physical setting is as vital as the quality of his/her food.

The best boundaries are those that establish firm ground rules for interaction with parents and family. The world is for exploration on a full sensory level, but relations with people must have reservations. These reservations cannot be established by reasoning; they must be established by modeling (examples for imitation) and firm, no-nonsense physical enforcement of correctives if infringements on established boundaries occur.

The parents provide continual opportunity for new experience in the most natural setting available and allow the child to set his/her own pace of exploration. The most fascinating experiences for the child are nearly always those of the parents: the mysteries of cooking and kitchen gadgetry, the tools for making and repairing, an automobile engine or a sewing machine. S/he will explore according to the nature of his/her own exploratory tools, the five senses. Through physical encounters with the tangible world of things, the mind-brain structures its corresponding knowledge of that world. The parents do not try to engineer this learning because they know that learning is a nonconscious process that must simply be allowed to unfold.

A child's ears, like all his/her senses, are acute and far more sensitive than the adult's. The child is given quiet because loud noises are terrifying. S/he might like to listen to conversations on a radio, but the sound level must be kept low. Noise is one of his/her enemies, like any sensory overload. S/he needs great stretches of peace and quiet, particularly in a natural setting of grass, trees, flowers. S/he needs to be left alone to hear the world, especially things adults no longer hear.

There are no big or little events to the two-year-old, all is breathless excitement, awe, and wonder. His/her logical feedback system feeds back on anything and everything experienced, not just on what adults value or think good for a child. Adult values block openness; we place priorities on this and screen out that. But the child accepts without question, at least initially. S/he does not screen out unless taught to do so—and/or unless s/he has built screens trying to avoid anxiety.

The qualification to the child's openness is that s/he must always have the right to place value on his/her own experience. Take the problem of food as an example: The twelve-month-old is a wonder to behold at table. S/he still nurses, of course, so food is not critical. S/he explores food as s/he explores everything else. Always a part of the family context, the child sits at the table and tries everything at least once, including salt and pepper and the flower centerpiece. Any and every new spoonful of food offered or grasped is willingly, happily accepted—a great game. Eating is exploration of the world, just as exploring the backyard is. S/he bites into everything with pleasurable abandon. Half of these bites s/he may also happily spit right back out again, just as s/he spit out his/her sampling of the stick. The two events are quite equal in his/her mind because his/her intelligence is open.

The spit-out bite registers as "not edible," but this is not negativity in the adult sense. It is simply evaluation after the fact. The spit-out item is assimilated and accommodated by the brain computer, just as the accepted bite is, and brings its own subtle shifts in the whole schematic that the child is building about food. Experience is experience, and new experience brings about increased brain activity.

Certainly, the positive encounter, that bite of mashed potatoes perhaps, is far more likely to be repeated. The child will probably gobble more bites of potato while stopping at one bite of broccoli, but both bring about some shifts in the general catalog of taste exploration. Above all, s/he is learning to explore freely, without anxiety. The mother keeps this openness by never tempting the child with items that must later be restricted or blocked, such as sweets, which hypnotize the young taste buds the way television hypnotizes the brain. In order to give choices and keep his/her system open and flexible, she makes sure that the areas of choice are beneficial.

For contrast, look over at neighbor-mother, a creature of anxiety, reflecting her husband's anxiety and their mutual attempts to structure reality intellectually. Neighbor-mother is very much concerned over her child's diet. She plans a careful, vitamin-filled, mineral-loaded dish tailored to fit his/her needs. Let me call this child Sam, just to keep our models clear. Sam is placed in his high chair, his bib tied carefully around him, to be fed his special diet before the adults eat.

Sam, too, is open to experience, being in his exploratory stage. He, too, accepts his given world without question at least once. She spoons him a bite of the dish, and he, too, accepts the bite happily; and as openly and happily, out it comes again. One of those mysterious dislike encounters has occurred. Sam's mother is patient and concerned; she carefully wipes up and offers him another bite. Again, he accepts it; and again, out it comes. Not-for-eating is his evaluation, but his evaluation is ignored, and around we go again.

After a few repetitions of this, concerned mother gets a bit aggravated; after all, she is the mother, she does know what is good for him, and this food is good for him. She is also conscientious; she reads everything she can get hold of about nutrition and tries to follow the welter of contradictions. She is also aware that he may develop a taste for the rejected food if she is persistent. And finally, she is irritated by his bad manners. Nice people do not spit out food, and it is never too early to learn.

The result for poor Sam is stalemate. His mother keeps insisting, and before long, he will not open his mouth at all. He ends in tears, is given a bottle, and is put in his crib so that the adult meal might get under way. After enough repetitions of this kind of encounter, Sam will no longer open his mouth for anything new. He grows very negative indeed. As soon as he has the language for it, he will automatically say "I don't like that" at the mere *sight* of anything new to eat. This will infuriate his father and exasperate his mother because it is patently illogical of him. "How do you *know* if you don't *try* it?" they all but snarl through clenched teeth.

At this point, Sam is using a shallow, one-dimensional world view as his criterion. He has constructed an arbitrary value system operating through one sense only: sight. He is using the great synthesizer of all the senses as a buffer between himself and experience, at least in this one aspect of his world. This blocks that total sensory information around which feedback can construct an accurate knowledge of the world. He has already, sadly, become like his parents, although they may never recognize this and although their resentment will mount over seeing themselves so blatantly duplicated.

Both children, the magical child and poor Sam, have formed a value system. The magical child's system is open-ended. S/he will enter into any experience without question, because s/he knows that s/he can return to the known without question; that is, should a new experience prove distasteful, s/he knows that s/he has the option to withdraw. Therefore, s/he is willing to enter into experience without judgment. His/her open intelligence arises from a sense of personal power.

Surely the child has no conscious awareness of having the power of decision. But his/her body has learned that s/he can enter an unknown-unpredictable and not get stuck there. S/he can choose to leave, but leaving is only possible by first entering. So his/her great learning is that one values experience only by entering into that experience. S/he does not learn to value experience before having that experience, which immediately restricts intellect to what s/he has already experienced and declared valuable or what offers enough similarity to a good experience for his/her long-range senses to screen, evaluate, and clear.

You may be thinking: Ridiculous! He must learn to evaluate, and ahead of time. He must learn to tell the difference between good and bad, right and wrong, and so on just to survive physically in the world, and this is our job.

I can only agree—with a qualification: But when? When is such evaluation preceding experience appropriate to the mind-brain system, to the tools of logic within that system? *Not in this most prelogical state of practical intelligence, when nothing is important except physical interaction with the world.*

No reasonable parent would feed a toothless, nursing infant great wads of steak, no matter how nourishing that steak might be, for the infant would have no tools for assimilating and accommodating to that tough meat. The parents of the magical child know that the nutrients of his/her mind-brain growth follow this same qualification. They know that to force the prelogical child to adopt the stances and attitudes of adult logic (or even the logic of a six-year-old) is specifically damaging.

Let's extend the child's ventures beyond that all-important family table. S/he toddles outside and stumbles into a mud puddle. Interesting stuff, this. Immediately, s/he does what s/he is impelled to do: S/he interacts, using all sensory tools in order to gain a full-dimensional knowledge of this particular bit of world content. S/he squashes toes deep into its nice, soft texture, scoops up a handful, feels it ooze deliciously between fingers. S/he smells the strange newness of it, stares at it long and randomly. S/he likes its texture and tastes it for identification, richly smearing his/her face in the process. S/he finds it not to taste, which his/her computer brain dutifully notes, along with all the other information pouring in for feedback reflection, cataloging, and relating. The stuff's tactile qualities seem to be its real element, and s/he explores this further. What possibilities! His/her concept of mud grows rich and full, lacking only a name label, which s/he will get soon enough.

Turn back to neighbor-child Sam and his anxiously conscientious parents busily splitting his natural wholeness into anxiety fragments. Sam, after all, is an attractive child, and they are sincerely proud of him. Mother practically lives to display her little possession to the neighbors. His new toddler clothes are perfect; he is ready for the photographer or grandmother. Little Sam also toddles out of doors. (His parents left the door open by error, and their backs are turned for a moment.) He, too, stumbles across a mud puddle—interesting stuff, this—and down he goes, as dutifully prompted by his intent. Nice, squashy texture, oozing between fingers. (Not between his toes, of course, for he is quite well shod in the proper high shoes to give his delicate little ankles all the proper support they need, the support that nature has so carelessly failed to provide, as every shoe advertisement makes clear.) Sam interacts with all available tools and eventually makes the taste test, too, leaving a wide swath of the stuff across his face, his two pearly front teeth now quite brown. He, too, decides that this is not pudding, in spite of appearances; but he, too, notices all its other possibilities—or starts to. For here comes mother. Horrors! Her little dear eating mud. All those germs! And his nice clothes. Suppose mother-in-law should come right now and see him. What would she think? What would she say? What kind of mother would mother-in-law take daughter-in-law to be?

Sam's mother is conscientious. She does try to keep him clean. She has seen, with a cringe, those pictures of little children with flies crawling on them, dirty, unkempt, in Bangladesh or wherever. She does carry her can of aerosol disinfectant when they go out, spraying a path of death before them lest some live organism chance upon her charge. Now here he is, wallowing in mud, even *eating* it. What perversity. What has she done wrong? She must ask her pediatrician. "No, no, *no!* Dirty, dirty, *dirty!* Bad, bad boy!" she wails, chanting rhythmic trinities as she snatches him up and rushes him off to the bathroom for a general purification.

Consider what happens to Sam's concept of mud. He cannot register any of the reasoning behind his mother's great outburst, but he surely registers her distress and anxiety. The whirlwind of action resulting is one long, sensory-overloaded blur, but out of it emerges one clear thing: Mud means trouble. Mud is *bad.* This trouble also feeds back in his logical computations of all this new information. But this negative business is not his own like-dislike evaluation; it is a surge of anxiety that makes no sense. He liked the experience, yet mother's reaction was so negative.

He is driven both to take his cues from her and to interact with his world. But his world interactions have again threatened his bond, brought anxiety and censure. His bond has weakened, not strengthened, his world interaction. The only possible results are confusion and failure to process freely his new information as it is. He learns to view his world through conflicting values that pull him in opposite directions. His world fills with encounters that might at any moment create this storm of anxiety in his matrix.

What about Sam's like-dislike responses? He learns that these have no meaning, that he is not himself a source of value. In the long run, he learns that he has no value. What of his feeling of personal power? Obviously, it never materializes. He learns that he has no power of decision. What of his muscular-mindedness for entering into the unknown and accepting the stress of the unpredictable? His validity as a legitimate source of interaction has been denied him. But, bear in mind, he has learned *value*. He bonds to his mother, to her anxiety and her value. His natural instinct for taking his cues from her grows; whereas in natural development, it should fade as autonomy unfolds. Developing no power of decision, Sam is doubly dependent on mother's cues to decide for him, a dependency that will eventually shift to his culture's professionals and institutions, who stand ready and waiting.

Sam's driving intent is nevertheless to interact with his world and structure a knowledge of it. He reacts negatively to the negations blocking his drive, but the stress his own negation places on his anxiety bond proves too threatening, and he eventually capitulates. Before any interaction with the world, he will check his parents for their reactions, for their signals of approval or disapproval. In fast, acute, intuitive glances, he will read their moment-by-moment anxieties concerning his actions and reactions and their fears concerning events that might occur.

Slowly, a screen forms between Sam and his world. This screen is a value system based on parental anxieties. Finally, he no longer interacts, maintaining a flow of energy with his world; he only reacts according to his learned value system for prejudging experience. His long-range senses are utilized as barriers between self and world contact because that world carries potential hazards, which, in turn, carry potential anxiety reactions from his parents. His world view grows flat and shallow, and because his genetic intent is thwarted, his anxiety grows apace. He is slowly split between the pulls of intent and the anxieties of intentions. His body expresses this split through bad health; every germ lays him low. He is bonded to an anxiety that blocks the muscular-mindedness leading to autonomy. He will never bond to the world and will have no safe place to stand. He will nag and fret his parents throughout childhood and on into his quasi-maturity, trying to wheedle from them a safe space that they do not have. He cannot bear to be separated from them because without them he has no cues for judging the unknown and the potential dangers inherent in every new event.

The magical child is allowed open interaction, free of concern for value or utility. This is possible only because the parents assume responsibility for his/her survival. They believe that it would be better for the child to enter his/her inheritance with some physical damage than to remain outside it physically whole. Psychological damage can block his/her entry into the matrix shifts that are to come. They do not load him/her with concerns that can register only as anxiety. Because s/he is allowed his/her own evaluations, such power of decision gives a corresponding power to act, and s/he responds to the instant unfolding of the moment as it is.

The child, roughing in a world knowledge, wanders without rhyme or reason, and s/he plays. S/he has no goals other than the moment, and no other time exists. To the child the time is always now, the place is always here, the center is always "me." For this is the way a world knowledge is structured.

At the same time, the parents institute an underlying strata of order. They give him/her four walls of "thou shalt nots" that are reasonable, unvarying, and consistent. These boundaries mostly concern personal relations. S/he knows exactly where s/he stands in relation to his/her parents, what they allow, what they do not allow. S/he is not faced with ambiguity or indecision.

No reasons are used with the prereasoning child in the expectation that s/he will grasp adult logic. Reasons can fill their conversations with him/her, but not their communications or directives. If correctives are needed, they are concrete. The parent picks the child up firmly and removes him/her from the bounds of transgression. They let him/her know without apology that boundaries are to be observed. The single word *no* suffices if the parent is absolutely consistent in his/her own mind, free of ambiguity about his/her actions, confident, decisive, and expecting full compliance.

Firm boundaries give strength to the bond and clarity to those areas open for exploration. The child clearly registers the parents' power of decision and their confidence in their decision. S/he feels bonded to strength. S/he accepts their boundaries and restrictions without frustration or hesitancy because s/he is geared to take cues from them, and their decisions are in keeping with his/her intent.

Anger may nevertheless occur. Anger in the child results when s/he is thwarted in intent. Intent has no logic, only drive. Frustrated in his/her immediate drive (and s/he has no time except now), the child wishes to remove the obstacle blocking him/her. Anger thus subjects the child to a peculiar and nearly unresolvable stress. His/her innate anger reaction over restriction by a parent is this nonlogical desire to get rid of the parent as obstacles, to get him or her out of the way. Immediately, this very reaction touches on or triggers the child's equally great dread of abandonment. That is, if the child's anger were to succeed, his/her parent would disappear, and s/he would indeed be abandoned. Such a split between drives (the one for bonding, the other for exploration) creates unresolved stress that feeds back into the anger, until the state of anger eclipses all its origins.

So the child must learn that his/her anger cannot in any way upset the bond. When his/her drive for exploration clashes with the parents' responsibility for his/her physical safety or the order and well-being of the family as a whole and his/her frustration of intent flares into anger, the child must learn that s/he can express this anger without threatening the bond. Not that anger is to be encouraged in some free-expression, let-it-all-hang-out slackness. Emotions are not at stake; the bond is. The child must learn that his/her spontaneous reaction of anger as a kind of death wish toward the parents can be expressed *without* being realized. S/he must discover that mother will not disappear if s/he does become angry with her. The child's own anger is the most explosive force s/he knows, second only to mother's anger. S/he must learn that not even the destructiveness of anger can destroy or weaken the bond.

And it is just as imperative that s/he learn that mother can express her anger toward him/her without in any way upsetting the bond. It is impossible for parental frustration not to flare up. The child, living in the unconscious of the parent, senses every volatile emotion, no matter how incidental or even whether expressed. S/he interprets unexpressed anger as potential anger the parent holds toward him/her, and s/he interprets their anger as s/he does his/her own, as a desire to remove the source of the anger. To the child, unexpressed parental anger means that they are suppressing or curbing his/her own abandonment, his/her own removal. S/he may suspect that their anger is suppressed and hidden because the bond cannot withstand that anger expressed openly. His/her bond is then threatened, and anxiety will result. S/he will start dividing his/her energy between intent and the need to try to strengthen the bond. S/he will be all the more afraid to express angers and frustrations for fear of breaking a suspect bond, and a combination of bottled-up fear, rage, and anxiety will result.

So the mother expresses her momentary irritation freely and openly. She tells the child exactly when she is angry, why, and how angry in matter-of-fact, nonapologetic terms. She then immediately reestablishes the bond in every way: by holding, body molding, eye contact, smiling, and soothing sounds. A playful acceptance of the anger after it has been clearly expressed lets the child know that the anger is what can be made to disappear, that personal power holds sway even over that most destructive of forces. The most threatening of stresses then relaxes within the bond because the child knows that no power on earth can threaten the bond.

With this freedom from anxiety and confidence in his/her source of power, the child moves into an autonomy suitable to his/her stage of development. Soon s/he can leave the mother freely and enter adventures on his/her own because s/he is sure of power and absolutely certain that s/he can return to the matrix without question. S/he is, in effect, carrying the matrix with him/her, and the mother is free of direct dependency for longer and longer periods; she is never saddled with a clinging, fretful child.

The mother risks her child because she knows that she has no choice except to trust the life process. None of us can guarantee ourselves our next heartbeat, nor can we guarantee the child's. The need to protect the child without crippling him/her forces the parents to make decisions. Because the mother bases her response on the life process, not on some jury "out there," she exercises prediction and control within her capacities and relinquishes control to the flow of things when she reaches her limits.

She allows minor hurts if need be. She knows that the child must discover through sensory interaction the cause and effect of the principles governing the world. She avoids the temptation to use verbal commands or descriptions as barriers between the child and interactions. She will surely caution against fire burning, but if a minor blister must result from his/her insistence on sensory exploration of what she means, she will allow just that if it can be done within sensible limits. She will label the experience with the single word *hot* as a future cue, but she does this without loading the word with any value because the child would register that as an anxiety value.

Above all, she will not load his/her action with the guilt of "I told you so," which is an attempt to assuage her own guilt (something this mother does not suffer). Nor does she load him/her with preconceptions based on "next time listen to mother," which is an accusation of wrongdoing. She knows the child has done nothing but follow intent. She gives a value-free name label for his/her encounter, and she allows the child to make his/her own evaluations of experience through his/her own concrete learning. If she uses that word *hot* again in reference to some event, the child will take cues from her readily enough and without anxiety. Hot will take its place in the scheme of things as naturally as the bad taste of the gritty stick.

The world knowledge that is structuring within the child has nothing in common with adult world knowledge. The word *gravity* has no part in the biological plan; it is a cerebral kind of term. But "fall down, go boom" is the body's knowing about the world, a primary concept about world-person interaction. Gravity is an abstract theory of adult thinking, an idea about relations, not the relations themselves. The biological plan needs the actual interactions between physical body and earth because that is how the brain hologram clarifies its picture of the world hologram. And (as we shall see in Chapters 16 and 17) the creative logic that opens at age seven can unfold only out of this concrete body-knowing. Abstract ideas about any of the child's world relations are not appropriate at this stage and are specifically damaging if given to the child in the expectation that s/he can incorporate them into his/her logic.

The period of roughing in is the great period of language development. The child is one passionate query: Whazzat, Mamma? Whazzat, Daddy? S/he rushes about in his/her excited exploration, pointing, asking for a name for every item s/he encounters, every phenomenon s/he experiences. The name given in answer to the question registers in his/her mind-brain as one of the concrete properties of that thing or event. The name does not stand for the event. The name is in no way distinguished in the child's mind from the thing or event itself. The name enters into logical feedback as a component part of the event, exactly as its smell, taste, touch, and sight do. The name becomes an integral, structural part of the brain's concept of that thing or event.

Remember that the newborn infant synchronizes body movements to speech used around him/her, that adults still mirror speech in micromovements, and that each person has a distinct repertoire of such synchronizations. Speech is a body process to the child, particularly during this roughing-in period; it is a body-knowing, no more learned than breathing or seeing. Speech is completely concrete to the child, directly connected with the tangible physical world, which includes his/her body.

Ask the two-year-old to say the word *hand,* and s/he will move his/her hand as s/he says the word. Ask the child just to speak the phrase *sit down* without moving. S/he will sit down as s/he speaks the phrase. Word and act are synonymous to the child because speech is a concrete body process, a physical response of musculature. Just as his/her brain structures its concepts by internalizing physical interactions with the world, the brain incorporates speech as part of this process.

Speech has no abstract qualities to the child, and his/her mind-brain cannot process information extracted out of the concreteness of his/her actual world moment. His/her brain can process only what registers through tangible sensory experience.

This concreteness of language holds throughout childhood and must still be acknowledged in the eight- or nine-year-old. Alexander Luria relates an experiment that clearly shows both the power of speech as a body coordinate and the child's inability to process abstractions. Three- and four-year-old children were given a rubber bulb to press whenever a light came on and release when the light went off. The task was simple enough, but the children were unable to do it, no matter how many times they were instructed or how the instruction was devised. So the experimenter started shouting "go" when the light went on, at which point the children squeezed the bulb correctly. The word *go* coordinated their body response to the light stimulus.

Then the experimenter had the children give themselves the signal "go" with their own voices when the light went on; the coordinations took place splendidly. They synchronized their muscular response to the light stimulus through the mediation of their own commands.

The next part of the experiment is even more vital to this discussion and gives insight into a critical problem in parent-child relations because it clearly emphasizes the child's inability to process abstract information. The experimenter tried explaining the experiment to his next group of three- and four-year-olds. He told them how to approach the problem; he gave simple, clear directions (showed them the bulb to press and the light to watch, told them when to shout "go" and how to respond to their commands). The children were completely incapable of responding. Then he made a much more detailed and thorough explanation, with examples and models, carefully rehearsing the operation for them. Again, they were incapable of following the instructions. No matter how varied, ingenious, and clever his instructions, each experiment failed when he gave the children their instructions in abstraction, outside the immediate context of the situation itself. The children could only grasp the nature of the experiment and respond when he gave them their instructions one step at a time in the immediate context of the event itself. They had to have that rubber bulb in their hands to grasp the complexities of squeezing it, see the light go on with that bulb in their hands in order to make the connection, be told to say "go" at the instant of the light's actual flashing in order to complete the circuitry.

The reason is simple. The child's thought process *is* his physical action. When the child is not acting, he is not thinking, in the adult sense of that term. The brain patterns a new ability as the child acts out the new actions that ability requires. The new ability is first roughed in by a kind of muscular response; the completion of the various parts of the task fills in the details; then there is the practice that smooths out the connections and allows variations.

To make sense to the child, information, instructions, and demands for obedience must correspond to the child's available touch, smell, sight, and muscular movement. Once an activity is learned through instruction, the words of that instruction are internalized along with all its other movements. But this internalization can result only from an exterior sequence of muscular acts according to the cycle of competence. "From the outside in" is the rule, and as long as the parent also remembers appropriateness (that a maneuver must be in service of the child's intent), learning can be quick, efficient, and early.

So the mother of the magical child responds to "Whazzat, Mamma?" with the name asked for, no more, as many times as needed. She does not load the request with an encyclopedic dissertation in order to make the child smarter quicker than anyone on the block. She does not load his/her request with all the peripheral notions and descriptions that adults stagger under, all the semantic undertones and overtones that trigger our many anxieties.

Understand the distinction here: In daily life, she exposes the child to as much language as possible. Parental conversations are vastly over his/her head, yet appropriate. But in no way do the parents err by carrying this over into communications of a learning or instructional nature. When the mother uses words to instruct the child, she uses words in a straight way —no baby talk, yet no abstract adult talk. She keeps to words available to the child's concrete touch, sight, hearing, smelling.

She uses imitation for instruction or explanation as much as possible. She shows him/her, one point at a time, and then s/he performs that one point with the mother's physical guidance and any concrete words appropriate. The mother does not give two instructions in succession. She gives each point and goes through the acting out of that point with the child before proceeding to the next point. She never moves to the next point until the child has grasped the first with his/her bodily response. If she wants the child to learn to put on socks, she joins him/her in the roughing in of the procedure; their hands are together in the movements, one step at a time, with no quick movements.

The mother knows that a learned activity, connected with or initiated by a verbal command ("Put on your socks"), ushers in specific physical entrainments of the same nature as trying to get the child to say "sit down" without his/her actually sitting down. Once initiated, learned physical entrainments, such as putting on a sock when asked, must play themselves out completely. Once such a complex of coordinated movements has been conceptualized in the brain (learned), it can be enacted only as a completely interrelated coordination. The brain cannot break up the entrainment. To do so, the child would have to be able to stand outside his/her own action objectively, which is a logical action of a very high level.

For instance, the mother asks the child to put on his/her socks (now that s/he has learned how). She then notices that the youngster is busy putting on dirty socks when she meant the nice clean ones laid out on the bed. She cannot then countermand the first order in midstream ("Oh, no, put on these cleans ones here"), handing him the clean ones, and expect him to comply. This is not possible because the child's brain will not have been able to process the verbal information for much the same reason that s/he could not as an infant both suck on the nipple and focus his/her eyes at the same time. A new entrainment absorbs the total system. Once started in the learned chain of events, his/her system is locked into the directing of muscular responses in a manner so totally integrated that once begun, the entrainment must play its complete role. His/her brain cannot attend the other order because it has not processed the words.

The child will have to be allowed to put the dirty sock all the way on before his/her conceptual system is free to process something else. Even if s/he could comprehend the mother's countercommand, s/he could not reroute the whole complex of mind-muscular coordinations. Only when the first sock is on, dirt and all, can s/he hear what mother has to say. S/he must then be told to take the dirty sock off. (Of course, mother can explain then and show him/her the clean sock.) Then, and only then, can s/he follow the new command and take the dirty sock off, which calls for nearly as involved a complex as putting it on required. Only when the dirty sock is off is his/her system clear for the final command: "Put the clean sock on."

Three different commands will have to be given, one at a time and only after the preceding action has been completed. Complicated? No. The real problem is its very simplicity. We choose not to believe such care necessary because we are too care-less, in too big a hurry to observe appropriateness. The clash that damages the biological plan is the clash between adult logic and the practical intelligence of the child.

How long does a physical incorporation of language last? Throughout childhood. Although body language of this simplistic sort seems limited, it serves the child's need perfectly because that need is to structure a knowledge of the actual world, not of the adult verbal descriptions of that world or adult ideas about it.

Ordinarily, the child completes the roughing in of his/her knowledge of the world at about three years of age. His/her interactions have built a critical mass of these rough concepts. His/her logical feedback then begins to order this mass into some coherent form. His/her exploration of the world has been random and haphazard because the intent was for un-differentiated content without value. Now, with something like 80 percent of his/her concrete body-knowing about the world formed, s/he is ready to fill in the details of this rather scattered and unfocused world map.

Chapter 12

Filling in the Details

Watch the three-year-old walk into a luncheonette where all the counter stools are helter-skelter. S/he will want to straighten them out, put them in some order. That is what his/her logical feedback system has now begun to do with those helter-skelter concepts about the world that s/he has amassed in two years of roughing in. His/her drive for undifferentiated content now shifts toward a preliminary ordering of knowledge into rough groupings, even as s/he continues the drive to amass world knowledge.

This ordering out of chaos has its precedent in the stranger syndrome (which was noted at about six months of age), when the child's logic put together all available information about mother and ended with a stable knowledge of her.

The preliminary ordering at age three is concrete; it concerns the tangible effects of the immediate world, and the mother responds to the child's new need with a more formal structuring of physical boundaries, more routines, more order, along with increased openness for exploration. The passionate "Whazzat, Mamma?" continues as the building of a reference library of names continues. At the same time, a new kind of query begins: "Why? What for?" The mother knows his/her ability to process abstract reasoning is still years away. She knows the child is not asking for reasons in the adult sense and that adult reasons may, in fact, be quite inappropriate to his/her stage of development.

Remember the three- and four-year-olds trying to press the rubber bulb when the light went on. They could not learn at all from abstract instructions; they could only process references to what they could touch at the time.

What the child can process in response to the quest for why and how are answers relating to what touches him/her: his/her concrete personal life experiences and, not incidentally, his fantasy life (an issue discussed in Chapter 15). Because his/her language grasp is enormous by age three or four, a parent is liable to think that this gives him/her a logical ability to process adult verbal logic. By age four, the child's language structure, syntax, and general ground rules are essentially complete, but this is not at all the same as the logical structure found in adult thinking. The mother of the magical child knows linguistic competence precedes logical competence by years. Four-year-old logic is a world of its own. She responds to her youngster's queries with simple, concrete answers available to his/her logical grasp, which means available to his/her sensory contact or fantasy repertoire.

She is not betraying the child's intelligence or intellectual growth in answering the question "Where does the sun go at night?" with "Behind the trees to sleep." If s/he asks why the sun goes out at night, the mother might answer, "So we can see the moon and stars." Half the children's stories handed down are fantasy answers to such questions.

The truth or falseness of the mother's answers or explanations are not always the primary concern. Appropriateness to the child's current state of logic is a more important issue. The mother knows that radical shifts of logic will later reorganize every meaning now forming in the child's mind. If s/he wants to know where the sun goes at night, the mother does not launch into a dissertation on planetary motion. She responds to the child's practical intelligence and his/her need for order and a logic of relations. These groupings are quite temporary. The purpose is not to grasp adult reasons, but to learn to form groupings of experience that make sense in the child's prelogical world. These are exercises of his combinational logic, and the exercises must use the tools of mind and materials available.

One "falls down and goes boom" and skins a knee. The force of gravity and the principles by which things hold together are understood quite well *as* skinned knee, the ball falling back down, the marble going down the drain. Around age seven, the child's creative logic, able to interact with and change aspects of the matrix, will develop out of his/her body-knowing the fact that "fall down goes boom." His/her body-knowing that fire burns and hot means don't touch will never need articulating for the unfolding of his/her miraculous logic lying in store. His/her body-knowings will be the materials out of which and on which his/her first great movements of abstract thought will be based because the growth of intelligence is from the concrete to the abstract, not the other way around.

To the child between three and six or so, everything simply *is*. Adult criteria and child criteria have almost no points in common. (Can't you remember being seriously puzzled over adults buying smelly cigarettes and such things instead of using all their money for candy, ice cream, and milkshakes as you would certainly do when you were grown?)

The mother does not impose criteria that are appropriate to a later stage of development on her child and so never questions his/her statements. The statement's content is another matter. If the child reports that s/he saw an enormous tiger in the bushes, she accepts his/her statement. The fact lies in the statement, not necessarily in its content. The truth or falsity of the statement is a different issue and very seldom the one to be dealt with. For example, if s/he says s/he saw a snake in the bushes and they live in the country, the child just might be making a different order of statement.

You may exclaim, "Aha! Here is contradiction. If you want the child to construct a true knowledge of the world, how can you possibly avoid teaching him the difference between childhood imaginings and the way of things out there in the tooth-and-claw world?"

These are good and sensible objections. In an age of crumbling social order, where even basic survival has become doubtful, how could one argue with such questions? Part of the issue is when and how are such issues learned and brought into practice. I am appealing for observance of a certain order of unfolding in the child and an appropriateness of materials. If our century has taught us anything, it should be that we cannot legislate ethics. The child's problem lies, not with such high-level qualities, but with the far more fundamental and approachable problem of adult-child interaction. The issue is that adult reality experience is a different order of logical structuring from child reality. The other part of the issue is that child reality needs no correcting by adult reality; it needs only the chance for proper maturation.

Adult experience is not of the one-for-one correspondence with the world that the child knows and has few points of similarity at all with the child's fantasy or reality. Adults view the world through an elaborate web of propositions inherited from ages past, unconsciously adopted as they grew up, rigorously learned in school, and all assumed to be absolutely true and necessary for reality adaptation, survival, and social acceptance. Adults see the world through this complex grid of abstract ideas in much the same way that the child sees his/her reality through a web of fantasy play.

When we realize that our concepts organize information into perceptions regardless of the nature or source of those concepts, we then realize how thoroughly our experience changes as we structure abstract notions about the world later in life. Our current state of affairs is always the result of our current set of ideas about things, our body of knowledge. Our current reality is always the expression of our ideas superimposed on the world as it is. World plus idea equals our adult reality experience, which we come to think of as the world itself.

We have no final way of being sure what a child's actual perceptions are, any more than we have for each other as adults. Perceptions are the end results of concepts, and concepts change. But we do have clues to the child's world perceptions. The art of children between the ages of two and six is remarkably alike all over the world.[1] After age seven, a child's drawings begin to show an increasing and decided cultural influence and so vary widely.

Perception is not a very accurate index of what is out there because different perceptions can form from the same source of stimulus and the same perceptions can form in people in response to different stimuli.[2] Surely we can look in the bushes to see if a tiger might happen to be there, but we cannot reconstruct the child's interior conceptual context of that moment to find out what was going on.

Imagination means creating images that are not present to the senses. All of us exercise this faculty virtually every day and surely every night. Illusion, fantasy, hallucination all fall into the same category of verbal explanation and explain nothing at all. These terms lead us away from, not toward, the key issue.

Stimuli can be elicited within the brain's own huge network of concepts (for the rhythmic firing and patterning almost never ceases) and can produce perceptions that have no external source.[3] As we grow older, we learn (or presume we learn) which of our experiences are legitimate indications of what *is* out there. About our only criterion for this distinction is consensus, and this opinion is what we learn as our culture's body of knowledge.

The issue of childhood fantasy and imagination will be discussed in Chapter 15 because the whole crux of human intelligence hinges on this ability of mind. Here it is enough to say that nature has not programmed error into the genetic system and that the child's preoccupation with fantasy and imagination is vital to development.

Frances Wickes relates the story of a nine-year-old child brought to her in serious psychological difficulty. He was confused, disoriented, extremely fearful, unable to attend school, unable to learn or take part in any ordinary life. His parents were well-educated people who had given their child every advantage, stimulus, and nurturing—to their best knowledge. They were practical, no-nonsense people who were determined that their child should not be saddled with the wealth of silly nonsense that seems to plague most children. They were scrupulously honest and never lapsed into any of the convenient and lazy social lies with which careless parents fend off their children's queries. They did not respond to questions of birth with stork tales; they explained carefully the full mechanism of reproduction and birth, complete with pictures and diagrams. There were no cheap fantasy tales of Santa Claus, fairies, or guardian angles at night. They chose the literature to be read to him with care, making sure it was sensible and informative.

He responded splendidly: an articulate, sober, thoughtful, and precocious child. His conversation at five was astonishing. But things began to come apart when he was about seven. Progress seemed to stop. Kindergarten had been a failure; he had been unable to be separated from his parents, and the situation grew steadily worse. He had serious night terrors and grew thin and frail. Finally, a childhood schizophrenia was the sad diagnosis. After a year or so of unsuccessful attempts at treatment, he was taken to Wickes, who settled down to find the root of the trouble. She gave the child the lead and took her cues from him, as children had taught her to do. Diagnosis took almost no time at all, and Wickes's prescription was a shock to those most literate and sensible people: Read to this child, she said, hours and hours a day. Read him nothing but fantasies, fairy tales, wild imaginative stories. Throw in all the talking animals, cloud castles, little people, magic and mystery, signs and miracles, Santa Claus and angels, fairy godmothers and wonderful wizards. Saturate him with the unreal and improbable. Make up stories for him, and enter into fantasies with him. Talk to the flowers with him, converse with the trees and wind, animate every nook and cranny of his life with imaginary beings.

Within a few months, the child was well, in school, catching up, healthy, and happy. Growth of intelligence had stopped around five because a vital ingredient was missing. Now the missing piece of his developmental machinery had been filled in or perhaps simply allowed to operate as nature intended: a way for ordering into meaningful relations a rather meaningless and haphazard world.

The child's need is to be a child. Forcing upon him adult thought produces a form of premature autonomy, even when that adult thought is cast in terms the child can grasp. Surely we can trick the growing system into walking before crawling, but that young system will reel about drunkenly and crash headlong—to the amazement and heartbreak of those parents so delighted that they had produced a child wonder.

So the mother of the magical child does not question her youngster's reports of private perceptual experiences. She knows that she has no direct access to what that experience might be, and she knows that her responsibility is of another order entirely, that she must not apply adult criteria and judgments to the child's perceptions. Her child's perceptions are always the truth.

If the four-year-old cries out in the night that there are bears under his/her bed, the parents accept that statement. His/her tears indicate not only a genuine perception to that effect but also, more importantly, specific needs that lie beyond the issue of illusion. The mother does not go in, flip on the lights, and berate the child for being silly and imagining nonsense. She does not insult his/her system and accuse him/her of being a fraud. Nor does she just cuddle the child and tell him/her everything is all right. Things are obviously not right. She does not show him/her that there are no bears under the bed. Instead, she recognizes the youngster's terror as loss of personal power, loss of control, some inarticulate fear projected onto an object of imagination, and fear that has an object is tangible and can be attacked. The child's matrix needs reaffirmation, particularly at this period of a division of labor taking place in his/her brain system. When this reassurance is needed during the day, which happens continually, s/he simply rushes in of a sudden to embrace the parent, be picked up, and hugged a bit.

The mother plunges to the heart of the matter; the bear *is* the focus. Immediately, she does that for which the parent is designed; she functions as the matrix. She lends her child her power. She gives her child the strength to enter fully into the reality s/he has created, and she joins him/her in that world. Together they get rid of that bear. Perhaps she holds the child and charges the bear and chases it completely away. Perhaps she corners the bear and cows it into submission. Or perhaps, holding the child, they make friends with the bear, win from him some boon, and make of him a guardian for future nights.[4]

She has not turned on the lights to prove her child a liar, to show that his/her perceptual apparatus is faulty. She has not tried to override the child world with the idea system of the adult. She has met the child where s/he is, in his/her need, taken her cues from him/her, and responded according to the needs of the situation. Rather than trying to dispel the reality creation, the mother has joined in transforming it. Personal power has overcome powerlessness and the fear of the unknown.

The child finds that the matrix has augmented him/her, given power, and made him/her larger than the opposing and challenging forces. The issue was not to try to change the context in which his/her perceptions had formed and so change the nature of those perceptions, which is what would have happened if the mother had turned on the lights. The light she turned on was in the child's mind; a learning took place.

To have demanded that this prereasoning child agree with and reflect back to them their own set of abstract adult reasons not only would have forced on him logic inappropriate to him but also would have created a form of psychological abandonment. The parents would not have met him/her where s/he is, the only place where s/he can possibly be, but would have retreated to a semantic-rational world beyond his/her capacity for response and meaningless in the situation. They would have isolated their child with his/her fears, even though they might temporarily calm him/her enough to allow them to return to their warm beds and forget the incident. And no learning would have taken place.

Chapter 13

Division of Labor:
Birthing a Self

Somewhere around age four, a majority of children experience nightmares.[1] The general theme of these bad dreams is separation from or loss of the matrix. Such a loss or separation threatens the child with a collapse into chaos because the matrix is the brain's conceptual orientation to the world. The nightmares are accurate signals, though, because at this stage a shift begins in the brain that will separate that child's functional awareness from the matrix functions that furnish his/her world. The long birth of *individuality* has begun and will be complete only around age seven.

Developmentalists agree that the social self seems to have its beginnings as a separate awareness somewhere in the third or fourth year, when egocentricity begins to fade. And all agree, indeed there is historical precedent, that this social self becomes fully functional somewhere around age seven. Any mother knows that her child has displayed a continuous, unbroken personality from birth; the uniqueness of each child is apparent quite early. But the child's own awareness of that uniqueness and corresponding loss of egocentricity are developmental, and are products of logical maturation.

In nature's economy, the creating of a unique and personal self depends on and is part of many biological processes. Individuation is also the means for, and is dependent upon, a division of labor in the mind-brain system. This division of labor is a slow process that begins only when three things come together: completion of the roughed-in world view; completion of the *corpus callosum,* a late-developing organ of the brain; and another brain-growth spurt, which always heralds a new era of stage-specific rapid learning.

In this process, the mind-brain will be divided into three interdependent and synchronous functions, each processing (and/or creating) information according to its functional needs: consciousness of one's self as individual, as unique, and as separate from the world; consciousness of one's body in physical rapport and interaction with the living earth; and consciousness of one's total hologram effect, of the life system in its total thinking sense, what Carl Jung called a *collective consciousness,* James and Huxley called *mind-at-large,* Deikman of Langley Porter calls the *general field of awareness* (my favorite term), and what the ancient Chinese may have meant by the *tao,* the flow.

After age seven, the functions apparently relate to specific areas of the child's brain; that is, particular areas of the brain begin to specialize. Social-self functions appear to orient to the left hemisphere of the brain; body-knowing and earth rapport relate to the older-brain systems; the primary process, or general field of awareness, orients to the right hemisphere. These functions are undifferentiated during the first three years or so because the total brain is engrossed in its single great task of structuring a knowledge of the world (as outlined in Chapters 11 and 12). No specialization between the hemispheres is feasible in this initial stage because the hemispheres are largely separated from each other. They are connected to the old brain, of course, and participate equally in the massive piling up of world concepts triggered by that old brain with its driving intent and muscular maneuvering of the body into interactions. When the child is about three or four, about the time of completion of the roughed-in world view, the corpus callosum, a huge network of hundreds of millions of nerves connecting the right and left hemispheres, completes its growth. Once this bridge of communications becomes fully operative, specialization of the two hemispheres is then practical. (Some specializations, such as using one hand dominantly, start in that second year, when the first functions of the corpus callosum can be found.)

The brain-growth spurt occurring at this stage-specific time prepares the brain to learn to relate and coordinate the three systems that are slowly differentiating. The process is slow because the logic of differentiation involved is enormous; the process is also part of the general ordering into coherency and filling in of details of the roughed-in world view. Logic is also preparing for the eventual practice of that completing world view, which occupies the fifth and sixth years, and in turn prepares for the great shift of logic and matrix at age seven.

The basic world view concepts have formed in the brain as a whole. As a result, no matter how specialized some area or organ of the brain might become later, this basic set of concepts will be the glue holding the parts together, the reference point or concept matrix. These concepts are concrete patterns concerning the actual stuff of the world, and out of this matrix, all future concepts must be generated, no matter how abstract and purely cerebral.

Around age four, this undifferentiated character of concepts and awareness begins to be affected by the logic of differentiation, and egocentricity begins to fade. The child's awareness begins to sense itself as an "it" separating from that matrix. Although the separation is only a functional one taking place in the brain, it is as real as the separation that occurs at birth, just much longer and more gradual. If bonding has been weak or conditional, the child undergoes an unconscious trauma, an anticipatory kind of birth stress, expressed in nightmare.

Egocentricity was not some illusion on the part of the early child or an error of brain functioning that adults must correct. Egocentricity clearly stated the case. The brain as a hologram is representative of the earth. So long as this is undifferentiated, the personality, or consciousness within that brain, receiving its perceptions from that brain, is literally an undifferentiated part of the hologram effect. It is part and parcel of the world system, which, because it radiates out from the child, places him/her at the center of thought, with the world a body extending from him/her. The clarification of the hologram (to use that model) is a period of breathless wonder and excitement for the child because s/he is discovering his/her larger self. Some objective awareness of the hologram may begin in that second year when the corpus callosum beings preliminary functions, but the first signals of this objectivity, which requires some separation, certainly occur around age four.

It is risky to use left- and right-hemisphere specializations as a model for the separation of self and primary process functions. Attitudes and theories about the differences between left and right brain will change with continued research. I use the model because it fits so well, but I ask that the functions I am describing be salvaged in case the model for representing them becomes obsolete. Our error would be in thinking that *mind* is the social self, our ordinary awareness, or any of the other functions. Mind and consciousness (at least ordinary consciousness) cannot even be equated with certainty. We know that consciousness arises from an area in the midbrain, not in the right or left hemisphere. Furthermore, both the old brain's body-knowing or earth consciousness and the (possible) right hemisphere's primary process are conscious functions in their own right.

Ordinary adult awareness should almost surely be a neat balance among these three functional systems because they are right here in our heads. We should be aware on a body-earth level, a primary process level, and a social-self level. The early child is conscious on a body-earth knowing level; the late child and preadolescent should develop (among many things) a fully objective social self; and the adolescent and adult should develop full consciousness of, and relationship to, the primary process, the general field of awareness. Each stage of development should enhance the previous stage. Growth is designed to incorporate more and more, not continually lose the unfolding levels of consciousness.

Adult conscious awareness cannot exist except in synchronous relationship with body-knowing and primary process. Yet we largely lose our child awareness and apparently never develop awareness of the primary process. The brain always operates as a gestalt, yet as persons, we seem stuck in one segment of the operation, that intermediate developmental stage of social consciousness. We adults get only very rare glimpses of these other two parts of our mind-brain, even though it is impossible that they not be equal parts of the function of awareness. Classically, we have referred to our ordinary, rather isolated awareness as real or normal consciousness. We have called any awareness of the other two functions *altered states of consciousness* and have been conditioned to believe them pathological aberrations. There are people who manage, through rigorous and lengthy disciplines, to become consciously aware of the primary process, that general field of awareness apparently embracing all thought everywhere. Reports of awareness of the primary process are referred to as "introverted mystical experiences," unity experiences in which no sensory activity is involved. Reports of consciousness of body-earth knowing are generally referred to as "extroverted mystical experiences," unity experiences of the hologram on a sensory level.[2] Although these altered states are largely denied validity by the academic community, they are so rewarding that people devote years of their life or risk their bodies and brains through drugs to attempts to experience them. Most of us border on falling into awareness of these other functions continually, which our conditioned social self feels to be a threat of a collapse into chaos because our idea schemes would apparently be overwhelmed. Yet the child mind is equally all these states. The child is all this without differentiation, though while conscious *as* them, he is not exactly aware of them, which is rather like a fish not being aware of water because there is no other world.

To become aware of the mother as a person to be related to and loved, the infant in utero must separate from her. To become aware of the infinite possibilities of the earth hologram and primary process, the child must separate from them in order to relate functionally to them. Among the many purposes nature has for the division of labor is giving the child this objectivity and distinction between possible functions. As importantly, only through a separated consciousness can a volitional, decision-making function be developed. The early child has no volition; the child's decisions are made by his/her driving genetic intent. (This is why it is not possible for the early child to disobey willfully.) Age seven has historically been called the *age of decision* because the objective self system becomes functional at this time.

If a mature creative synthesis were to act on our basic world view concepts, we would lose our orientation, live in chaos, and not survive. So some portion of the brain system must maintain our initial, and accurate, world orientation. Naturally enough, this is the job of the old-brain system. It replicates the brains developed over millennia for relating to the earth. The old brain actually runs the body, from first heartbeat to last gasp, maintaining the body's homeostasis (stable sameness)—the synchrony of heartbeat, oxygen content, blood pressure, glandular output, body heat, the coordinating of quadrillions of cells—a job carried on without our conscious awareness and, thank God, without need for our volitional interferences.[3] The old brain is probably the carrier of our genetic coding, providing the single driving intent that propels the infant body into interaction with its earth, so it is only economical that this system maintain our primary world view in the original structure developed and perfected in the first seven years.

The primary process is the function through which we are conscious of the earth as a thinking globe, the flow of life, the general field of awareness, and almost surely, even larger ecologies of thought. The primary process is also past, current, and potential possibility and experience. Other cultures have maintained a much greater openness to the primary process than Western culture has, but some university laboratories are beginning to get minuscule glimpses of a possible bridge. Since the primary process is the general field of awareness, it also encompasses the earth hologram and so is closely linked to the old-brain system. Indications are that the right hemisphere (which has traditionally been connected to the left hand) is more intimately connected with body processes than the left hemisphere, lending some support to using this as a model for primary process and social self. Through biofeedback, we are making rudimentary moves toward strengthening ties to the older-brain system; but unfortunately, we are using biofeedback to try to seize volitional control of autonomic processes that are not designed for such control. In focusing intelligence on such an arbitrary interaction, we fail to see that harmonious synchrony with old-brain functions, not volitional control of them, is the issue. Having so little awareness of our primary processes, the next thrust of our alienated efforts at control will be to try to seize volitional control over primary processes, which will further fragment intelligence. Yet, our ordinary consciousness cannot help but be the result of all three functions, a paradox that has filled many volumes of speculation.

The division of labor is designed to develop a gestalt self, a conscious, volitional awareness able to orient to the living earth exactly as it is; creatively interact with that earth through creative logic (a logic that can interact with the hologram to change aspects of that hologram); creatively interact with the mind-brain's own products, which include the primary process; and finally mix the three capacities.

Each of these capacities is also a matrix, and the developmental stages being outlined here are the structures and shifts of those matrices. The first seven years are spent in structuring a knowledge of the earth as matrix, and the self must then be born out of that matrix in order to relate to it. This relationship is the development of personal power and creative logic, which give the self as the new matrix at adolescence. Standing in that matrix, mind then structures a knowledge of the primary process and becomes matrix itself, completing the movement from concreteness to abstraction.

Nature would never program our automatic shifts of matrix without also programming adequate bonds for us between our matrices, just as the infant at birth has its umbilical cord and a host of other channels for interaction with the new matrix. The great shift unfolding at age seven is every bit as critical as the one at birth. Unfortunately, it virtually never succeeds; virtually all of us were stillborn at this birth.

Understand that the separation I am talking about during the period from four to seven is a functional separation within the brain, a separation between the earth hologram effect in the brain, a conscious ego system, and a primary process. The bonds to be established are signals, functions, patterns of rhythmic firing of brain cells, processes of interaction within the brain. The primary process proves to be the bonding agent, an agent which is then designed to expand into its own full dimensions as eventual matrix. Because the bonds between child and earth matrix are established through the embracing primary process, I call them *primary perceptions;* for all bonds are perceived experiences. Primary perceptions become noticeable (if we bother to notice) around age four, along with those nightmares, brain-growth spurt, completion of corpus callosum, and all the rest.

Chapter 14

Primary Perceptions:
Bonding with the Earth

"I see white light coming out of your head and fingers," reports little Jessie. "There are bright colors around your face and body." Larry, aged seven, sees white light moving in and out of people's bodies. He sees red light around trees and orange light around dogs. Brynn, seven, sometimes sees specks of color float around her bedside. So go the reports from children studied by James Peterson. Over the past two years, child psychiatrist Gerald Jampolsky has studied some 150 children, who, between ages three and four, have also reported extrasensory perceptions.[1] Jampolsky's cases fell largely into classical extrasensory categories: clairvoyance, in which events taking place beyond the range of vision or hearing are reported by the child; telepathy, in which information or messages come from specific people at a distance; precognition, in which an event is perceived before it has actually taken place.

Considerable literature exists on ESP and psychic phenomena among children. Eloise Shields presents evidence that telepathic ability peaks at age four, at which time their parents may begin to be aware of such activity.[2] An English acquaintance of mine, who considers herself psychic and who can certainly pick other people's brains remarkably well, told me that her two daughters displayed astonishing psychic abilities at age four. These abilities proved to be in the ESP categories, with telepathy between mother and children being the strongest. Sadly, the abilities faded by age eight, a source of chagrin to the mother.

While working on materials for her dissertation, a musicologist friend discovered that almost any four-year-old child has perfect pitch (the ability to recognize and name musical sounds). All that was necessary was preliminary work with them in labeling so that they could communicate their knowledge and an explanation of what the game was about. She found, however, that the majority of children lose this ability by seven or eight.

Already the ramifications go off in every direction: Why age four? Why do such abilities so often fade at seven or eight? Do all children possess such abilities? If not, why not? Can these abilities be encouraged? Are they worth encouraging? Of what use could such capacities be?

These talents are biological, part of nature's built-in system for communication and rapport with the earth, part of our bonds with that matrix, part of the emerging system for survival, related to the division of labor, almost surely stage-specific in their unfolding, and no more fragile or rare than general intelligence. I find no evidence of being without a vehicle of expression; we cannot experience any phenomena without an operational structure for organizing that content into a perception. No matter how abstract, ethereal, or remote a phenomenon might seem, so long as we are here in this quite material body, that effect must be structured through our conceptual system.

I prefer the term *primary perception* to extrasensory perception because all perceptions of this nature must arise from that primary process within us. I have a number of examples that I favor because of their authenticity and clarity. Some of these I have used in a previous book, but confess that I now see them in a more practical framework.

Dr. Charles Tart relates an experiment in telepathy in which a person was placed in a sensory-isolation chamber (a room from which light and sound are excluded). The person was then connected with a polygraph machine, and he was covered with electrodes to pick up all brain-wave activity (EEG), monitor his heart and pulse rate, record muscular activity and sweat, and so on. All these readings were recorded by the polygraph machine, giving a rather thorough indication of what was going on with that person. A considerable distance away, in another isolation chamber, another subject was going to be periodically shocked. The first subject was asked to try to sense when the second subject was shocked. The first subject never seemed to sense when the other was shocked; telepathy was apparently not increased by isolation. But that first subject's polygraph reading showed significant leaps at the precise instants that the other subject was shocked.

Why, the researchers wondered, did subject A not know when subject B was shocked, when all of subject A's body readings clearly indicated the exact moments? Obviously, the self system, which subject A thinks of as the whole show, is only one of our concept-percept processes. Ernst Hilgard, of Stanford University, in his twenty-odd years of research into learning, trance, and hypnosis, finds evidence of different learning systems and even different perceptual systems within each of us. That with which we identify as anxiety-conditioned adults is only one part (though I am sure a major part) of our complete thinking organism.

For a couple of years, friends and I met regularly to delve in amateur, haphazard ways into the latent possibilities we had sensed within us. We learned to enter a deep hypnotic state by suspending all volitional control over personal body movements and thoughts and surrendering our volition and decision making to a member of the group. One evening, when it was my turn to act as guide, I had prepared some geometric drawings, carefully made with compass and ruler. I had these in a manila envelope, and when the group reported the required hypnotic depth, I explained that I was going to look at some drawings to see if I could telepathically send these images to the group. Everyone agreed on the purpose (agreement being a necessity), and I pulled out the first drawing, a kind of square cross inside a circle. I had thought it would be necessary to concentrate very hard and long in order to send the image, but before I even had time to take a good look, everyone "had it." Spread out around the dimly lit room, flat on their backs, with eyes closed, they indeed had seen or perceived each image almost simultaneously with my own looking. At no point did I do anything; indeed, I seemed incidental to the process.

A naturalist specializing in the study of foxes described his long-term study of a particular fox family located near a creek in a ravine. One beautiful, sunny afternoon, he observed the mother doing something he had never seen a fox do. She suddenly left her burrow and kits, went up the hillside some thirty yards, and began busily digging another burrow. She then carried each of the kits up the hill to the new den. Several hours later, the reason for this atypical act became clear. Although the weather remained beautiful and clear, a flash flood cascaded down, flooding the ravine; a cloudburst many miles upstream proved the culprit. Had the family remained where they were, they would surely have been drowned.

The newly developing science of earthquake prediction relies heavily on clues furnished by animals. Shortly before an earthquake, domestic animals become nervous, fowls refuse to roost as usual, burrowing animals leave their holes, rats and mice leave buildings.[3]

Primary perceptions are bonds with the earth, the natural interrelations of the hologram. A primary perception may take place through, but is not limited to, the five senses. In the early years, primary perceptions are almost surely part of the general cognitive fabric of the child's reality. Not until some division of labor among brain functions has begun and the effects of selective inattention have encroached will primary perceptions be distinguished by the child as something other than his/her ordinary five sensory functions. Primary perceptions are as biological as any other form of perception; are almost surely genetic to our species (as well as many other species), rather than space-age esoterica, spiritual gifts, or psychological aberrations; and are (or should be) clearly developmental, as all intelligence is. Furthermore, ESP is only one manifestation of the primary process from which such perceptions arise.

Primary perceptions are biological because they take place within the mechanism of the brain. We cannot perceive anything except through our conceptual processes. We all know people who believe themselves above material and mundane things or who partake of universal, spiritual capacities. *Always,* they, too, have, at base, those mundane biological functions of brain operating, although those operations may have expanded wonderfully beyond our mundane practices. Recent evidence shows that some so-called psychic phenomena, in which objects are moved by thought, relate directly to the old brain and cerebellum—and for good reasons.[4] That is where all movement is coordinated, where our concrete world concepts remain intact, where brain hologram and earth hologram mirror each other. There original language as a body response remains intact, and word as label and the object so labeled remain a single unit. The old brain is not personal as such; it moves deep into our material grounds of being. Psychokinesis (or moving objects by thought) is quite rare before age seven but is frequently found (increasingly today) after that age. The reason is clear: Psychokinesis is a creative interaction with the earth ordinarily stage-specific to the shifts in logic and matrix taking place then.

On the other hand, primary perceptions such as ESP are simply matters of information selectively drawn from the flow of things through the individual primary process in one's brain and communicated through ordinary conceptual patterning. No creative interaction or acting back on the earth matrix is involved and so almost surely different brain functions would be employed than in psychokinesis. ESP is simple reception from the primary process, designed to enhance well-being and security and to give information over a wide range. When the Ugandan mother intuitively knows her infant is about to urinate, she is not relying on ordinary conscious decision making except in responding to her signals; one way of describing this is to say that her right hand responds to and carries out the orders of her left hand. Bonding is one aspect of primary perception, whether at birth, or at age seven, when we should bond to the earth. Fragile and tenuous at birth, these bonds are designed always to grow into channels of personal power and possibility.

Although all brains are patterned alike, probably no two of them have ever functioned exactly alike. The possibilities for rhythmic patterning among those billions of neurons in the new brain are simply too vast and flexible for us to point to one area as *the* area for some activity. Rhythmic patterning changes continually, enlarges, shifts. Where primary perceptions such as ESP form, I do not know. Because they do not involve movement, they probably do not involve the cerebellum. Furthermore, brain function and thought product are probably never exact equivalents. Brain and thinking may operate like conductive wire and electricity. The brain may conduct but never actually contain thought, just as the body may have energy flows and rhythms that operate in conjunction with it, rather as the radiation belts operate around and yet within the earth.

White finds that approximately one child out of every thirty is exceptionally bright, happy, socially charming, versatile, flexible, physically healthy, and adaptable in outstanding ways. He also finds that this development is anything but an accident. These children have enjoyed surprisingly similar home environments and parental interactions in spite of sharp differences in social, economic, and racial backgrounds. His findings call to mind the sharp difference of intellectual growth between the Ugandan child delivered at home by the mother and the child delivered in the hospital.

In the same way, there can be little doubt that primary perceptions are the birthright of each child, just as superb intelligence and happiness are. Most of us, after all, are born with a pretty standard huge brain. Even when damaged, the brain's ability for compensation and recovery is remarkable. However, more children display ESP than superb overall intelligence, indicating that primary perceptions are so much a part of our genetic fabric that they are even less prone to destruction than other aspects of intelligence. This means that our built-in capacity for bonding with the earth on a physical level is powerful and more tenacious than the more fragile capacities for developing high-level abstract thinking and creation. Certain kinds of ESP have frequently been observed in mentally retarded people, again indicating that these capacities are part of our built-in machinery.[5] This also indicates one of the probable causes of the loss of such capacities. The mentally retarded cannot be fully acculturated (anxiety conditioned), channeled, and restricted the way the rest of us can through social cueing that shuts off primary perceptions.

Primary perceptions are developmental in that they tend to disappear, like a muscle atrophying, if they are not developed along with the rest of our faculties. They must become part of overall logical development, continually reinterpreted according to maturation. Logical maturation should act on the conceptual structuring of primary perceptions, just as it does on all learning, and these capacities should grow accordingly. Our perceiving of the primary process is always subject to our general conceptual ability. A primary perception suddenly breaking in on the awareness of an adult long out of touch with this aspect of life would be as disorienting as vision flooding the system of the congenitally blind. As a result, once our primary perceiving has atrophied, our self system develops a kind of defense against any such disorientation, locking us pretty tightly into our social consensus.

The primary process is ordinarily quite selective, drawing on the field of awareness according to the needs of the particular individual. As physicist Robert Jeffries pointed out several years ago, telepathy most often takes place between persons with close emotional ties. Telepathy with one's own child is therefore quite easy to establish and develop. Jeffries suggests that a family practice telepathic communication right before sleep and right after waking, starting with simple targets and working toward complexity. Again, the problem is conceptual: learning to pattern information from the primary process, learning to cue properly and attend the often subtle forms the perceptions take.

By selectivity, I mean the kind of attending found in Dr. Tart's telepathic experiment. Subject A's primary process gave clear body signals of the moment when subject B was shocked. Out of the multitude of possibilities within the general field of awareness, the process chose according to the request made from the individual self system, even though that self system did not know how to open to the answer. Here again, we find the real thrust and meaning of individuation and its role in the hologram possibilities of life: The unique and separated self, with its volitional system and capacity to choose, selects some target from the primary process, or plays with some possibility out of a continuum of possibilities (see Chapter 15). The primary process responds to volition and furnishes the result. Dr. Tart requested certain information; the primary process responded with clear perceptions.

Shortly after one of my sons turned four, I noticed his interest in and aptitude for music, so I started him on piano studies. He sat in my lap at the keyboard, I placed his hands on mine, and we "did notes." I used little verbal instruction, but we sang our notes as we played them. With one hand, we pointed to the note on the page; with the other, we played the note, switched hands as needed, up and down, rhythmically swinging through page after page and then book after book of "little fingers" music, one-note-at-a-time stuff, which was just my speed. Before long, I simply took my hands out from under his, and he was doing notes, singing descriptions, swinging along. It was fun. For the first year, we played together that way; then autonomy took over, and he sat alone. By then, he had left my one-note stumbles behind, and I placed him with a Julliard graduate who concertized in our area. By age five and a half, he could read almost anything his hands could encompass. He had perfect pitch and wrote tunes while sitting in his window seat. He would sing them to us, go back, harmonize them in neat classical triads, go to the piano, and play his finished piece. By age six, he played Bach, Clementi, and Bartok with astonishing skill, ease, and sophistication. His hands coordinated perfectly, his sight-reading was superb, and he memorized almost immediately. His teacher and I could never understand how he knew classical harmony intuitively, nor how any of his skill had unfolded so rapidly.

By the time he was seven, however, he faltered. We had started him in private school at five. He quickly became a fine reader and an all-round splendid student. And the more he became immersed in reading, to the great applause of parents and teachers, the more rapidly his music collapsed. By eight, his coordination was gone, his superb reading ability was gone, he no longer had perfect pitch, and he no longer wrote pieces.

A number of factors had entered at age four: The rudiments of individuation had given the possibility of creative relations between self and primary process. Our extremely close rapport had given a mutual exchange, our own form of psychological communication. In spite of my lack of keyboard skill, I had extensive musical study and experience. All this had acted as a strong stimulus to my son's similar leanings. The primary process shared between us had this immediate continuum of possibilities on which to draw. His learning was kept completely within the category of play, and because that play involved, for the first year, actually sitting in my lap, the entire venture took place in the safe confines of the bond. Performance or learning was not the issue, stress and anxiety were avoided, and so he learned at a remarkable rate. He played, and the absorbent mind characteristic of that period worked beneath the surface, exactly as the two systems, play and work, are designed to do. (In Chapter 18, I will explore how this synchrony is split by schooling, in which the self is not allowed to play but must try to do the work, wrecking the marvelous balance of forces involved in learning.)

Primitive peoples often exhibit a fine sense of balance between volitional choice and primary process in their learning. Farley Mowat, a Canadian biologist, relates the story of how an Eskimo friend of his, the "minor shaman" Ootek, gained an uncanny knowledge of and rapport with wolves.[6]

Ootek's father had been a full shaman (a kind of spiritual leader, medicine man, and mediator for his people, who communed with the spirits and rulers of nature). When Ootek was five years of age, his father left him with a wolf pack for twenty-four hours. After an initial thorough sniffing, the adults ignored the child, but the cubs played with him, roly-poly, the entire time. Then the father returned, walked into the pack, and retrieved his son. As a result of this experience and the general tutelage of his father, Ootek could interpret all wolf calls for the tribe. For instance, at one point, he heard quite distant wolves howling, then a nearby pack answering the distant signals. Ootek announced that a caribou herd was so many hours north, heading west. The hunter of the group immediately left, returning the next day with ample meat, having intercepted the caribou just where Ootek had indicated. On another occasion, Ootek heard distant wolves, delightedly leaped up, and excused himself to prepare for a short trip. The wolves had informed him, or rather he had eavesdropped on their signals, that people were some certain hours away, heading toward Ootek's camp. Ootek knew, somehow, that these were his cousins and, according to proto-col, hastened to meet them. The next day he returned, happily introducing his cousins to Mowat.

We have no way of telling when primary perceptions begin to function, and we have a tendency to lump all sorts of nonordinary phenomena under a handy heading such as ESP. Actually, a wide range of intellectual capaci-ties are involved. The selective capacity of the absorbent four-year-old mind to draw on a continuum of knowing, as I am sure happened in Mozart's case (he never attended a day of school) or my son's case, is one of the myriad possible uses of this synergy and only by degree different from mother fox knowing a flood was imminent. Telepathy is just such a commu-nication between individuals through the primary process, and it begins to be noticed around age four.

On the other hand, imaginary play projections begin very early in the child, as do visual phenomena later lost to us. Around fifteen months of age, most children begin to point.[7] In the home, pointing may be a request for a name. In most cases, the child points and then watches the parent to read the parent's body and facial reactions. Outside the home, in a park, for example, the child uses pointing in a highly stylized manner. In his/her explorations, s/he moves away from the mother but nearly always remains within sight of her. When s/he encounters an unknown or unpredictable event, s/he stops, turns partly toward the mother, points to the unidentified phenonenon or event, and looks intently at the mother's face. S/he does not speak or make any sound. If the mother smiles, s/he moves to interact with the event. If she frowns, the child immediately returns to her. If she pays no attention or makes no response, the toddler will go to her, tug, point, and watch her face. Anderson, who spent a great deal of time researching this pointing syndrome, says that many times the child, on receiving no response from the mother, goes to her, tugs, points, and when s/he still does not get a response, finally verbalizes: "Man coming," or "dog coming," or perhaps using some general animal name. The frequency of this phenomenon intrigued Anderson because neither he nor the mother ever saw the various people, animals, or things toward which the child pointed in these cases. Anderson referred to these as the child's "imaginary novelties."

To the very early child, primary perceptions would be indistinguishable from any other experience. The child is biologically geared to take his/her cues from his/her parents. Only as the child begins to sense that the parents do not take part in, share, or approve certain experiences can s/he possibly begin to differentiate among his/her own perceptions. In this, we have one key to the all-too-frequent failure to develop primary perceptions. Part of the two-year-old's passionate "Whazzat, Mamma?" is the desire to have his/her experience verified. This reality check with parents occurs throughout childhood. Pointing serves the same purpose, and in the open, it serves (or must once have served) specific survival purposes. Infant animals newly taken into the field by their mothers follow much the same procedure as the pointing two-year-old.

When a child gets his name label for an experience, the name enters into the concept concerning that experience and becomes an integral part of the thing-event's structure. In addition to being a mind-brain-body coordinate, the name gives the child a common ground with his/her parents concerning that experience. They have granted sanction to that experience. The child will then selectively attend this kind of experience in the future and be much more likely to repeat it, filling out and practicing that particular concept. Furthermore, his/her shared experiences reinforce the bond with the parents and continually verify his/her increasingly selective experience and world view.

If the child asks for a name and, for whatever reason, does not get it, the child senses that the parent does not share that experience or give it sanction. The concept of that event will not be filled in; it will remain shallow and eventually disappear. Selective inattention results.[8] When a child reports some phenomenon that the parent has no grasp of, as many of Jampolsky's and Peterson's children did, the parent is usually disturbed. This negativity is immediately apparent to the child and weighs against his/her repeating the experience. Sooner or later, the child's concern for bonding, and later his concern for social consensus, will lead to selective inattention, screening out that kind of experience. Peterson showed some older students pictures drawn by his seven-year-olds showing various odd colors around things and asked them if they had ever seen such things. "Yes," they replied, "but not anymore. Caused too much trouble." And it had taken Peterson some time to win the confidence of the seven-year-olds so that they would confide in him all about the colors and things. They all had said that when they told their parents about it, their parents' *colors* changed—to red.

The problem of imaginary perceptions in children has long been a subject of discussion and debate, just as their general magical thinking has been. The psychologist Smythies once spoke of the "quasi-hallucinatory character of childhood." *Hallucination* is an interesting term: "a pathological manifestation . . . a pictorial and symbolic expression of neurotic mental structures." Because childhood in all cultures is filled with such activity, we must then assume children are born with quasi- or partially pathological or neurotic mental structures. Of course, we straighten them out.

Hallucination is any perceptual phenomenon not shared by whoever is setting the criteria or making up the terms. (That is, agree with me, or you are, by definition, crazy.) Virtually all children in all cultures share this failure to distinguish between the real and the nonreal, which would indicate, according to our terms, that nature has somehow programmed error into the plan.

Some people might feel that my examples of nonordinary phenomena and exceptional children do not represent the norm and so are not valid. Had White simply observed that one out of every thirty children was exceptionally bright and made no further investigation because they certainly were outside the norm, we would not have the fine insights he has given us. But he moved to find out why, and he clearly shows that the exceptionally intelligent child receives a very specific (obviously exceptional) kind of interaction with his/her parents.

In the same way, to consider ESP a rare gift is to miss the significance of our whole heritage and take the easy way out. There are no errors programmed into our biological plan. Primary perceptions are bondings to the earth and no more rare than the infant-mother communions observed in Uganda. Such communions are not found in our country simply because we treat our infants differently and so we get a different product.

Think of ESP as the primary perceptions becoming functional around age four, when the biological division of labor has begun. Active associations and relationships of a perceptual nature can begin the exchange between primary process and child. The logic of differentiation is then beginning to distinguish between self and world. Only then would any particular otherness of a primary perception be noted. Examine the character of the perceptions these children report. They note that a person's color changes according to mood. Consider clairvoyance, precognition, telepathy. Do you not see how vital such capacities would be for the general bondings to the earth as the child prepares to move from mother toward the wide world?

Primary perceptions are designed to establish links between self and world, and they utilize sound biological procedures in the brain. Primary perceptions furnish a way of drawing on nature's body of knowledge and of being informed by this general field of awareness as needed for well-being. Consider Ootek and the wolves; the fox mother and the flood; animals before an earthquake. Do not be too ready to dismiss the implications here, for we are dealing with a 3-billion-year genetic system that can code almost anything into a brain. Although we have alienated and estranged ourselves so thoroughly from our larger body of life, as Dr. Tart's experiences show, that larger body and marvelous heritage have not abandoned *us*. Unless perfect pitch is explained and enough roughing-in instruction is given for the child to be tested for it, the talent will never be perceived. Could this not be the case with many other talents vital to our well-being?

Shields finds telepathy peaking at around age four; most children lose it somewhere after seven. Van de Castle finds a decline of extrasensory perception in general by the seventh grade.[9] Should telepathy peak and fade? Should my English friend's little girls have lost their capacities around age seven or my son have lost his gift at that age? Should my musicologist friend find perfect pitch at four but not at seven or eight? Should the infant's ability to recognize the mother's face fade within a few hours after birth and not be reclaimed for weeks? Should the infant's initial excitement so quickly turn to distress? Piaget finds a form of creative logic unfolding in late childhood that he calls the highest form of human intelligence, but he laments in noting that the ability is almost never found in adults.

We observe all sorts of marvelous qualities unfolding that then disappear, and we assume that they were simply passing aberrations and so *should* disappear. Some people respond that my examples are not typical and so not valid. From where are they taking their models? From the lowest common denominator after the damage has been done, just as Spitz and the rest assume, over and over, for generations, that the newborn should be a vegetable because Freud said so.

Chapter 15

Play:
In the Service of Survival

Play is the universal characteristic in the young of all higher species. Because the economy of nature rules out random or wasted action in the formative period, the child's driving intent to play all the time must logically be a major part of the biological plan. Piaget found that play was "in the service of intelligence" but *not* developmental; that is, play serves many vital needs and functions of the child's growth but is not in itself a source of conceptual growth. Intelligence grows when the child encounters some new information or event, assimilates this into his conceptual system (just as we digest food), and makes an accommodation to that event (just as we grow new muscles). Accommodation means structuring new conceptual patterns in the brain to account for the dissimilarities in the new experience or problem. Previous patterns grow more flexible through accommodations, giving a greater ability to interact. Intellectual development always involves a balance between the ability to assimilate and the ability to accommodate. Play, Piaget says, is not developmental because this balance does not take place. In play, it is as though the child can eat and eat without anything ever reaching his digestive track.

Two categories of play are observed in the child according to Piaget: *fantasy play* and *imitative play.* Both forms use imagination, which is defined as "creating an image not present to the senses." Fantasy play is often called *symbolic play* because a form of symbolism seems involved; that is, an object becomes symbolic of larger, more realistic phenomena. In fantasy play, materials or objects from the world are assimilated by the child and interacted with, but the child's conceptual system makes no accommodation to the object. His/her fantasy interactions are that the objects s/he interacts with do the changing.

The child sees an empty matchbox. This matchbox offers a whole continuum of possibilities for that child's imagination. The matchbox with its cover off can immediately be seen as a bed, a boat, a car; with its top on, it becomes a chest for treasure, a cash register. An inner image or idea of the possibilities inherent with that shape is projected onto the box, the box then becomes, for example, a boat. The box does not stand for a boat in that child's play reality. The child's actual concept of boat and his/her concept of box make no adaptation to their marked differences. The child's brain dismisses all dissimilarities the box actually has to the pattern of boat. No rerouting or relaying of the points of dissimilarity takes place in his/her brain. The child's image of play overrides the differences. The inner image fills the gaps between the established concept of boat and the information coming in from the box. The brain assimilates the sensory stimuli of the box, but only those points of similarity held in common with the inner concept of boat are used in the fantasy perception of the child's play reality. The mind-brain clearly distinguishes the play reality from the world as it is. When the play is over, all concepts remain as they were because only imagination was used to fill the gaps in the rather astonishing dissimilarities. Thus, there is no development in the ordinary developmental sense.

In fantasy play, the child registers stimuli from part of his/her world. S/he takes in an object, but s/he makes that object accommodate to him/her. S/he makes the object serve his/her fantasy image by transforming it to match that fantasy image, and his/her play is with that transformed object. The child has, at this point, bent the world to the service of desire, as Piaget expresses it.

In imitative play, there is no assimilation, only accommodation. The structural change that takes place is only in the child's bodily movement used in the imitation, not in the conceptual structures of knowledge about the figure imitated. The child observes some particular physical activity in a parent, for instance, and mimics those actions with his/her own. For instance, watch a child observing the father shaving. The child will move his/her face in the particular grimacing motions the father makes. The child watching the mother mix a cake will go through the same motions as s/he watches and will repeat these motions when given pots and pans to play with. This imitative play is obviously useful for learning immediate social rules and practical actions; it will take on greater significance after age seven.

In imitative play, the child acts as though s/he is the adult model s/he is imitating, and the purpose of the imitation is to assume the powers of the adult imitated. The game is to accommodate to the model by adapting one's own body to the actions of the model. The more perfect and accurate the resemblance of body movements, the better the play. For instance, when I was nine or ten, we would come home on a Saturday from the Tarzan movie and feel impelled to strip down (no matter how cold and wet the weather) and go leaping from branch to branch of the little apple tree, making appropriate ape calls, beating our chests as our hero model had done. By our physical accommodations to his image, we were ourselves then transformed into that image. And in that transformation, we assumed our model's powers over the world. In fantasy play, the box became the boat; in our imitative play, our spindly shanks and chests were transformed into the glorious power of the ape man himself. The image out there had transformed the image in here.

Thus, imitation serves the same function as fantasy play: The child plays that s/he can exercise a control over the world, bend that world to some desire within, or that s/he can become the desired model, with all that model's power, by imitating the model's actions. The central act of mind in both cases is imagination. Imagination is possible only to the extent that the conceptual patterns from which points of similarity can be drawn are there in the mind-brain system. The object must offer a continuum of possibility, and so must the brain's knowledge. A child can only imagine him/herself to be someone else or one object to be another when both subject and target exist in his/her structure of knowledge. The boat is not present to the senses, only a little matchbox; Tarzan's muscular prowess is not present, only skinny limbs. But a sufficient number of points of similarity between the actual object (our skinny limbs) and the internal image (our knowledge of the model) *are* present. The points of similarity are sufficient for the conceptual image held within to fill in the gaps created by the dissimilarities and so create the necessary reality perceptions that make up play.

Filling in the conceptual gap with imaginary material, ignoring all dissimilarities, is the essence of child play. The regulatory feedback mechanism apparently makes a clean distinction between the imaginary filling in of the gaps of dissimilarity and the actual reroutings necessary by an actual concrete interaction. The concrete concepts of the world are kept separate and so not changed by these incomplete acts of play. The great rule is: Play on the surface, and the work takes place beneath. The child's mind plays on the basic conceptual brain set without altering it, rather as a musician plays on an instrument without his play altering the character or nature of that instrument.

As I have noted, growth of intelligence is never a conscious process; conceptual changes always take place below awareness. Of what is the child aware in fantasy play? S/he is aware of the reality of his/her own play creation, a reality that exists neither in the world out there nor in the concrete concepts of the child's brain. Play reality, like adult reality, is neither world nor mind-brain; it is world plus mind-brain.

How many times have we heard parents and teachers complain, "All they want to do is *play*"? A child's relentless absorption in play seems to be a problem for adults. Nearly everything we want to do to, with, and even *for* the child seems to run against this formidable competitor. Play and *reality adjustment* are counterclaims on the child. His/her intent is to play with the world; whereas our intentions are to make him/her attend ideas of ours and work.

Psychologists have found a relationship between animal play (particularly among higher primates) and human play. In both, play offers a way by which the young can learn the social rules and adapt to them with minimum risks. In both, play offers a chance for the child to learn to use tools without economic pressures. Vigotsky gets close to the matter in his observation of play as a "pivot between the real and the imaginary." But he misses the point by not understanding the difference between world and reality. Almost unanimously, psychologists fall into the error of considering the child's play to be wish fulfillment at a fantasy level.

Because play absorbs the majority of a young child's life (and on into adulthood) and is an incredibly varied and rich activity, almost any comments about it are in some way probably applicable. Beneath all the studies and comments about animal and child play runs a central, if unrecognized, thread: Play serves survival. But our notions of survival are so grim, so opposite to play. The very word conjures up pictures of a gray, marginal existence, hanging to life by a thread, down to the last tissue or tank of gas. Instead, consider survival to be the victory of life over death, a cause for celebration. This victory is what constitutes most animal play, even such a purely economic function as the chimpanzee playing at termiting (extracting termites from an anthill by inserting a piece of straw into the entrance hole). Consider the passionate intensity with which young animals play; the abandoned joy and even frenzy with which a puppy leaps up at the slightest invitation, dashes madly about, ferociously closes in to snapping range, bounds away in great circles, works himself to fever pitch. He is practicing mock battle, perhaps closing in on the prey. In my play with him, I may be another dog with whom he is doing mock combat or some fantasy rabbit projected for his pursuit.

Animal play clearly serves several purposes: learning of social rules in a nonserious atmosphere where mistakes are tolerated, mock hunting if the animal is a predator, mock evasion if he is a prey animal, mock combat if combat is part of his species-societal means for establishing hierarchies, mock mating or preliminary sexual play before full sexuality emerges. All these are necessary to the animals survival learning.

The young rabbits in my backyard, being prey animals, play the exciting game of evasion: freeze, listen, move fast; freeze, listen, move fast; dodge, twist, leap, double back in random, haphazard, but purposeful enthusiasm. This is the practice of their survival, and such practice is always joyful for all species because one always *wins* in play (at least child play). Play is its own reality experience, a state in which survival is always successful, where life always wins out over death. The image within being projected without does not have to adapt to the actual concreteness out there; what is there adapts to what is within. The young animal glides smoothly into autonomy without ever making a distinction between the preliminary play and the later work.

And what of the child? The underlying purpose of the child's play is the same as those other species. There is a qualitative difference, though, between the nature of the animal's play and that of the human child. The difference lies in the nature of the child's fantasy and the thrust behind his/her imitations and the tools and techniques of survival being unconsciously learned.

I am sure no animal is aware that it is learning survival techniques as it plays with its mother and siblings. Surely a human child has no possible notion of survival learning, no more than the two-year-old is aware that his/her mind-brain is structuring a knowledge of the world. Intent always precedes ability; the biological plan prepares for functions that will become fully operative much later.

This brings us to an underlying hypothesis running throughout this book: the *dual* nature of the mind-brain. I am not referring only to a division of labor involving separate hemispheres and so on; I am also referring to two levels of activity that are going on in the child almost from the beginning. I have said that the first seven years are devoted exclusively to one thing: structuring a knowledge of the world exactly as it is. And yet, in the economy of nature, many functions are accomplished at once, and again, intent is always running years ahead. We find that "all they want to do is play," and the child spends virtually all his/her time (if allowed) at play. S/he is designed to play with the world, experiencing both the world and his/her play reality. The reality played with is the world filtered through the fantasy projections of play.

In the conscious awareness of the child, there is play. Although play is not intellectual development, as Piaget makes clear, every nutrient needed for structuring a world view can be furnished by play. The child's intent drives him/her to maintain the parental bond, explore the world, and play in it. When intent can express itself freely, no dividing line grows between any of these critical needs.

While the child plays on the surface, the great work goes on beneath. Regulatory feedback, conceptual construction, and synthesis, all the mechanics of learning, are nonconscious procedures. Awareness is the end result. We are always recipients of, not the manufacturers of. When the intentions we press on the child are in flow with his/her intent, s/he learns quickly and joyfully because then it will be his/her play with us. Interaction is play, but action and reaction are work. The biological plan is aborted when we invert this genetic plan for learning. That is, to approach learning consciously, we think we or the child must do the *work* of learning, but that is a biological impossibility. The greatest learning that ever takes place in the human mind—a learning of such vastness, such reach, such complexity that it overshadows all other learning—takes place in the first three years of life without the child ever being aware of learning at all.

If play is in the service of survival, does the child then play at mock combat, hunting, or evasion? Not at all. The child plays at imagination, creating images not present to the senses; or s/he plays at fantasy, bending the world to his/her desire, taking some object present to his/her senses and transforming it in his/her mind-brain; or s/he plays at imitating, becoming the hero-heroine model by imitating the model's precise actions and so assuming the model's dominion over the world. And what does every child believe every adult capable of doing? Of actually being able to bend the world to an inner desire, exactly what the child is busily practicing in his/her passionate play. And what does every child dream? Of possessing his/her own powers over the world when s/he grows up. And how are these powers developed? By the child's following his/her intent. And what is that intent? To play.

Animal play perfects specific survival maneuvers and techniques. These are ways of interpreting and responding to the environment by appropriate physical maneuvers. The child's play is also designed to perfect specific survival maneuvers. But the child's maneuvers are not physical; they are intellectual, the maneuvers of an infinitely open intelligence and an infinitely flexible logic able to mirror back a created image and change some aspect of the hologram within. This is what the huge brain is for, to go beyond the cause-effect confines of the hologram itself.

As the Duchess says in *Alice in Wonderland:* "take care of the sense, and the sounds will take care of themselves." The rule for the child is: Let him/her function, and the structure will take care of itself. Three things are going on in the formative years: His/her brain is constructing an accurate conceptual view of the world as it is; s/he is playing continually that s/he can change that very world; his/her experienced reality is a casual mixture of these two, which is another major reason for the child's long-delayed autonomy and another reason why the parents must assume responsibility for the child's survival. Survival play cannot give the child survival; only as this play merges with the work of the creative logic unfolding at age seven can the child learn to survive as intended.

The compelling nature of play poses a problem for adults wishing to get the child to attend to adult notions of reality. The child's intelligence becomes invested in his/her imagined transformations of self and world, and these are singularly compelling. His/her awareness locks into fantasy; reality becomes that play. For the child, the time is always now; the place, here; the action, me. S/he has no capacity to entertain adult notions of fantasy world and real world. S/he knows only one world, and that is the very real one in which and with which s/he plays. S/he is not playing at life. Play *is* life. As Piaget expressed it:

> [For the child] play cannot be opposed to reality, because in both cases belief is arbitrary and pretty much destitute of logical reasons. Play is a reality which the child is disposed to believe in when by himself, just as reality is a game at which he is willing to play with the adult and anyone else who believes in it . . . thus we have to say of the child play that it constitutes an autonomous reality, but with the understanding that the "true" reality to which it is opposed is considerably less "true" for the child than for us.

The mind-brain system is designed to maintain the matrix in its original form, even when it furnishes the reality experience of play in response to the child's intent. Such a sophisticated division of labor occurs almost from the beginning (play can be observed in two-week-old infants) and could only take place by careful genetic provision. And yet the overwhelming response —at least from educators and psychologists, and so seeping down into consensus—is that play is a kind of atavistic, primitive, animallike irresponsibility the child stubbornly insists on, a diabolical magic thinking s/he indulges in to try to avoid coming to grips with the real world and learning about the brass tacks of surviving. Analytical psychologists and behaviorists speak learnedly of fantasy play as wish fulfillment by which the child builds a bulwark between him/herself and the harsh realities of the world. The child, according to this learned theory, fantasizes to keep from facing the awful truth of human frailty, awareness of his/her impotence in this uncaring universe. Or fantasy play is viewed as a kind of psychological safety valve, allowing the child to ease the pain of actual existence by magical dreams of power over it.

Nothing of the sort is involved. The biological plan is vastly more intelligent and skillfull and the purposes of play and imitation are light-years beyond these paltry, facile, impotent, and deadly unimaginative academic ..otions. Play is not evasion of a grim survival necessity; it is in the service of survival. The animal's survival play centers on mock battle, hunting, evasion because these are the specific activities it will employ at maturity for its physical survival. The human child's corresponding activities are imagination, fantasy play, and imitation. These are the specific acts genetically provided for, imposing an inner imaginary construct (not present to the senses) on an actual concrete event of the world (available to the senses) in order to change the context of that event or the content of some aspect of the earth itself. The great shift of logic at age seven is to merge work and play. Then the conceptual structuring of the earth will be complete and no longer draw a line between the conscious play and the unconscious work when transformations are called for.

At no point should there be any break between the fantasy play of childhood and the application of that play through the creative logic unfolding at age seven. As Colin Turnbull points out, the African Pygmy child plays at adult reality throughout childhood, and the adults delightedly play with the child in his/her learning. And one day, quite easily and naturally, the child's playing merges with theirs.

When a line forms between child play and adult work, the interaction between human and earth collapses. We are then isolated with our own energies—and work we must, indeed. The problem set for us is not to try to turn back to aboriginal man; that is impossible. The problem, if we are to survive, is to erase the line between work and play. Only then is personal power amplified by the matrix.[1] With a technological human, the resulting power would be awesome and magnificent indeed, were s/he in a balanced bonding with the earth, and that may be the direction toward which the world is tending.

Part III

Transforming the Given

Chapter 16

Dancing through the Crack:
Operational Thinking

On the island of Bali, seven-year-old girls are chosen to be *trance dancers*. Immediately on being so honored, they join the older girls and women in rituals that include stately dancing over coals of fire.

Ernst Hilgard of Stanford University found that children become highly susceptible to suggestion at age seven. This suggestibility peaks around ages eight to eleven and fades around age fourteen. At seven, the child undergoes a brain-growth spurt and a dramatic shift of logical processing. Because individuality is just becoming functional at seven, the purpose of the new logic and the new learning capacity is to gain self-sufficiency or autonomy, independence, and the ability to survive in the world.

The seven-year-old is ready to learn how to interact dynamically with the new matrix, the earth, by means of his/her new logic; s/he is ready to learn that when s/he gestures to the earth, the earth gestures back, just as the mother did. Through interchanges of this sort, events beyond the ordinary concreteness of the earth can take place. Through such use and practice, the child develops the tools of logic now opening just as s/he developed his/her first tools and logic through interaction with the mother.

A knowledge of the world has been roughed in, and the details now begin to be filled in. These details are what the reality of world plus child can mean. The new logic is for the unconscious work of the conceptual brain, in balance and harmony with the world, to move in synergy with the conscious play of the new individual, although always on behalf of physical survival, for which play has prepared the child. Through interaction, the assimilation-accommodation cycle can complete fantasy plays previously left incomplete and make them real, the world bending to the inner desire as needed for well-being or protection.

The seven-year-old is designed to learn this bending of the world by imitating an adult model. When the child accommodates his/her body to the adult model, a full cycle takes place; his/her logic assimilates the act, and things begin to change both internally within his/her concepts and externally within his/her reality. In the new logic of individuality, creative relations can take place between the two systems in the brain (the world structure within the primary process and the self system). The brain hologram is now essentially complete, and it can reflect back on its larger earth hologram and relate creatively. Now world system and child mind assimilate and accommodate as an interacting unit of relations and produce events beyond the possibilities of either system alone. The only difference between the reality experience resulting from the new creative logic and the previous fantasy-play reality lies in the accommodations between earth and child. To the child, of course, play is play.

Piaget gave this logic the formidable title of *concrete operational thinking*. *Concrete* means what it says: the tangible world and its processes. *Operational* refers to a controlled alteration of materials (as in the operational rules of a game, operating a machine, or a doctor operating on his/her victim). In operational thinking, the mind-brain operates on its information and changes that information's structure. *Thinking* still means action for the seven-year-old (and does so up until age ten or eleven).

This rootedness in body action is the reason operational thinking is concrete at this stage. The new logic can organize only around and out of what the brain has at its disposal: the concrete concepts of the actual world, as structured in those first seven years. The brain system cannot accept or assimilate information that does not have a sufficient number of points of similarity with its existing conceptual system. Through concrete operational thinking, the child's mind-brain can operate on and make transformations of its incoming sensory information so long as that information is concrete.

Throughout the earlier formative period, concepts were constructed from the child's sensory interactions with the world. At seven, concepts can be constructed on creative ideas concerning that world. A concept based on an idea rather than on something of the world is an abstraction, and the kinds of abstractions the child's brain can assimilate at seven are those that can be drawn out of, or detached from, the concrete concepts.

During the first seven years, when accurate world structuring was vital, imagination did not become conceptual; the brain did not accommodate to fantasy ideas. The matchbox certainly did not become the boat as far as the world or that matchbox was concerned. The brain dismissed all dissimilarities and gave a play-reality experience that left the vital concrete elements of world orientation strictly alone.

At seven, the brain can construct concepts out of imaginative ideas or possibilities that apply to the immediate reality, and such a pattern then functions as any other concept does: as a pattern by which the brain puts together sensory information. An abstract concept based on an idea about something can put together the stimulus information coming from that thing. The abstract pattern acts on that stimulus according to the idea about its source rather than on its actual structure. And that, roughly, is how operational thinking operates on its incoming sensory information.

The Balinese child, by imitating her superiors, operates on her incoming sensory information and changes it. She knows, without thinking about it, that the fire will not burn her because she sees the other dancers and knows that they do not get burned. She knows that by imitating their body gestures, she, too, will have their powers over the world and go unharmed. This is what she has unconsciously practiced in imitative play for years. The difference now is that, with her new logic and new brain growth, her imitative movements bring about a corresponding concept of action patterns in her brain, as always and just as nonconsciously. Thus, she bends some aspect of the world to her desire, not by some intellectual knowing of how to manipulate information, but by the same kind of automatic work within her brain that makes all conceptual growth and change possible. Her system operates on the incoming information through a combination of patterns: those from the world of cause and effect and those from the idea system of her models. The individual piece of the hologram that is her brain, now functionally clarified and able to reflect the whole, can change some point of the total structuring. In the interaction of matrix and child, the matrix reflects the change and so moves beyond itself.

The child's sensory information must bring in reports of the fire, the flesh, and the effects of the two; that is what her primary world concepts and body-knowing are designed to do. However, this information is contrary to her well-being, and concrete operational thinking, having been given (through suggestion) a model for another possibility, follows suit and operates on the information, changing it into something more compatible. Her thinking bends the world out there to the inner desire not to be injured. All that is needed is for the child to furnish the function; her mind-brain furnishes the structure. The only way the function can be furnished is the actual physical interaction. The assimilation-accommodation cycle, which was missing in fantasy play, is filled in by the new logical capacities. The play on the surface and the conceptual work beneath it merge as needed or as opportunity arises.

To be appropriate to the needs of the child at this stage, suggestions given must have sufficient points of similarity to the concrete world immediately available to the child. The child's concrete concepts give an accurate knowledge of the world, an accurate orientation. But even as these concepts formed in those first seven years, her parallel fantasy played on this concreteness without in any way changing it. The pianist plays on the piano; a piano tuner operates on it and changes its structure, keeping it in top form and harmony. The child's conscious self plays on the world; logic and intellect operate on and keep the instrument, the child's body, properly tuned and in harmony with the world. The wonder is, both performers—world structure and child structure (mind-brain)—perform on the same instrument at the same time and in keeping with the needs of each. That is what the division of labor was about. The concepts of world organization formed by seven are inviolate; the playing has not changed the instrument. Furthermore, these primary concepts are the means by which communion with the earth and flow of energy are maintained.

To grasp how people walk on beds of fire, we must understand how concrete operational thinking involves a primary process that includes the world and its offspring, the person. The findings of biology and physics no longer allow the assumption that world and mind are separate elements. A world without thinking would have no life. It is thinking that creates a planet different from, say, the dead moon (assuming it is dead). There is no way to distinguish planet from its planetary life any more than there is to distinguish a live body from the life of its cells. Remove the life from its cells, and you have a different body. Earth without life would be a corpse. To assume that a relationship does not exist between the cells of life produced by the larger body of life is ridiculous. To assume that individual life can exist without accommodation and provision by the host body earth is ridiculous.

The examples given in Chapter 14 were of phenomena not possible without a general field of awareness or a hologram effect between earth and organism. The fact that this function is not available to rational academic thought hardly means that the effect is not there as part of the earth's processes. We did not know of the Van Allen radiation belt until recent machinery detected it, but the aurora borealis operated right along in spite of our ignorance. In the same way, evidence clearly points to the living earth interacting with her creatures, and the more complex the brains involved, the greater the possibilities for interaction.

The child's own experience and knowledge are only a small part of the information and possibility available through his/her primary process, but the conceptual set in his/her brain is the only means through which any of this potential can be made available to him/her. His/her communion with the flow of life must itself be grouped into meaningful patterns by the brain if volitional conscious interaction is to take place. Patterns for communion and interaction with the earth must be nurtured and developed as diligently at age four and again at age seven as such patterns with the mother were at birth, else they atrophy.

In the examples of the Eskimo and animals, I showed how their relationship with their environment included a range of communion beyond their long-range senses of sight and sound. In the same way, the child has relations with his world beyond sensory range, and these concern his well-being in the same way as those of the animals do. But no matter how clearly nature might signal, as with the fox on the river bank, the child must have the necessary receptors developed to receive and comprehend those signals. The only way these receptors can be developed is to be used, which means, of course, recognized and encouraged by parental nurturing.

The possibilities for creatively interacting with the world at age seven are of a different order of logic from primary perceptions. Perceptions are passive; we receive them. Operational thinking is active; we must do it. But, as usual, intent must receive its content from without. The possibilities for doing must be given the child through specific modeling in an actual situation that the child can imitate and so bring about the conceptual growth. The child's own imagination still gives only fantasy play, which never changes the conceptual world structure. The concrete concepts about the world can, of themselves, offer only the concrete world experience. Fire can, of itself, only burn. The world offers no abstractions out of itself. It has created the human mind-brain to do that.

To *grasp* an idea means to construct that idea formation in your brain. At seven, this can be done only by relating the suggested idea to the concepts that make up the child's brain patterns, which are concrete. S/he can grasp abstractions only if s/he can act them out in his/her immediacy. His/her thinking is still tied to action. To be appropriate to the needs of the child at this stage, suggestions given must have sufficient points of similarity with the world immediately available to him/her. Physical modeling by parent or guide is the way nature has designed learning for this period. Suggestions can be verbal if given one step at a time in the immediate context of the physical action, but modeling coupled with verbal cueing is far more powerful. Remember the children pressing the rubber bulb by shouting "go." Nature has provided that this body-language unit remain in force as a vital role in concrete operations. The Balinese child grasps the idea she sees by making the corresponding movements at the same moment. Her conceptual system patterns those movements because only by the patterns can the external movements take place.

Jane Belo, who studied the Balinese dancers years ago, was struck by the fact that the child could immediately execute the intricate dances with such polished skill.[1] Consider that the child has watched such dancing all her life (such rituals filled a large part of Balinese culture), that imitative play is a part of child life, and that physical movements can be roughed in just by watching.

Edmund Carpenter relates how eleven- and twelve-year-old inner-city children were taken to stables, shown saddle horses for the first time, and told they could ride.[2] The youngsters immediately rushed to the horses, leaped skillfully onto them, and rode galloping away with astonishing skill, just as they had observed hero models do on television for years. Those actions were thoroughly ingrained as a kind of empty category simply awaiting the chance to be filled in. (The fact that television is the most powerful influence on these children, as the cultural rituals are for the Balinese, is an issue to which I will return in Chapter 17.) When the Balinese child follows this same pattern in imitating her heroine models, she may also be simply filling in, with her new logic, patterns roughed in visually over the years.

A man came to a magical child seminar as the result of an experience that had unnerved him and threatened his academic and rational world view. His eight-year-old son was whittling with a knife, slipped and severed the arteries in his left wrist. Following an instant's panic at the sight of the spurting blood, the father, as if in a dream, seized his screaming son's face, looked into his eyes, and commanded, "Son, let's stop that blood." The screaming stopped, the boy beamed back, said "okay," and together they stared at the gushing blood and shouted, "Blood, you stop that." And the blood stopped.[3] In a short time, the wound healed—and the father's world almost stopped as well. He knew disorientation and confusion. He could not account for his own actions or the words he had heard himself speak, and he surely could not account for the results. He did not understand that the child is biologically geared to take reality cues from the parent; he did not know of the high suggestibility of the eight-year-old, of concrete operational thinking, or that at this age his son was peculiarly susceptible to ideas about physical survival. But some part of him *did* know and broke through in the moment of emergency. All the son needed, of course, was the suggestion and the support.

The creative logic unfolding during this late-childhood period can be summed up as *reversibility thinking,* an ability that Piaget calls the highest act of human intelligence but, sadly, the rarest. Full reversibility thinking does not unfold until adolescence, but its early concrete form is what the examples I have cited have displayed. Reversibility thinking is, to use Piaget's description, "the ability of the mind to entertain any state in a continuum of possible states as equally valid, and return to the point from which the operation of mind begins." A simpler statement would be: Reversibility thinking is the ability to consider any possibility within a continuum of possibilities as true, knowing that you can come back to where you start from.

This is what the child has been doing in his play for the first seven years. Fantasy play is entertaining a possibility from a particular continuum as valid. And always the child came back to the point from which the venture began; the matchbox was once again just a matchbox. Now, at seven, this play becomes a full operation, not just a fantasy reality on the surface of the concepts. The ability to accept outside possibilities means the ability to entertain them in the mind, assimilate them, and make an accommodation to them. A sharp qualification lies with the word *continuum.* A continuum is a logical grouping of those possibilities that fit. In fantasy play, anything can be anything else only within strict limits. The matchbox offered a specific continuum determined by the box's characteristics and the related knowledge in the child's mind. The matchbox could be a bed, car, boat, wagon, treasure chest, and so on, all transformations within its points of similarity. The matchbox offered little possibility for being a doll, animal, soldier, or rocket ship, but a clothespin offers just such a continuum.

An object that simply replicates something else offers nothing for this creative act. Creativity is precisely this capacity for seeing one thing in something else, seizing similarities and dismissing dissimilarities. At seven, this play capacity can become real if given the proper stimulus, although to the child, reality is reality. Any concrete possibility suggested to the child becomes valid as long as the idea is suggested by modeling and has a sufficient number of points of similarity with his/her concrete world knowledge; then the mind-brain can assimilate as his/her body accommodates by a proper imitating.

To entertain possibility, the child must be able to act on it. Ability depends on openness to ideas, which requires a certain freedom from the fear of the unknown-unpredictable; a sufficient number of points of similarity between the idea presented and the structure of knowledge; the flexibility of logic sufficient to restructure the dissimilarities (accommodate to the unknown-unpredictable elements), which is gained through practice; and the coordinating of mind-brain with muscular responses. The range of the body's physical capacities to respond enters into the range of general intelligence. The child's ability to synthesize and respond in this way is learned and developed by actual doing. If an idea or instruction given him falls outside his ability, he will simply be confused. Willful refusal is probably very rare because the child is geared to respond when the cues fit his stage of development.

At age seven, children have as passionate a longing for creative interactions and learning as they earlier had for explorations of the world. The mind-brain-body system *wants* to learn; that is what the brain-growth spurt is for. The longing this brings about is a drive, just as the longing genital sexuality brings about is a drive. Learning is a nonconscious biological process and will take place automatically when the models given are appropriate to the needs. In cultures where children are allowed to interact with adults, these children immediately imitate adult survival practices during the years from seven to ten or eleven. This is their play, and they develop great skill at it. The peculiar thing about culture has been that it takes the accidental forms of creative logic or reversibility thinking that occur and ritualizes them, turns these into religious acts instead of correlating them into a fabric of action. Such ritualizing happened on Bali, and among many Eastern cultures.

Many times I have been asked: If a child is not taught in the very beginning that fire burns, but instead is taught that fire does not burn, will s/he not then be able to walk fire from the beginning (in effect)? Such a notion involves a number of misconceptions. First, of course, we do not teach the early child in this sense; the child learns through physical interaction with what is. That fire does not burn is a contradiction and an impossibility for the world or the fire. Unless the little Balinese girl had a full-dimensional knowledge of her world, including the clear knowledge that fire burns if you touch it, she could not make the sophisticated abstraction that fire walking requires. In order to make a logical, controlled operation on the sensory stimulus of fire on flesh, she must have accurate concepts from which and on which the necessary abstractions can be drawn and built. A sufficient number of points of similarity between actuality and idea must exist. Reversing the ordinary cause-effect flow of life is possible only by having a conceptual pattern of that cause and effect.

Fire walking is such a common occurrence in so many countries simply because of the universal experience of fire itself. The idea is assimilated so easily because the points of similarity are so great that the few points of dissimilarity needing accommodation are not overwhelming. The act is impossible and incomprehensible to thinking *as* thinking, but not to thinking as action. Thinking as thinking can rearrange only abstract patterns in the brain, and fire burning is a very concrete pattern. The only way an abstraction can be drawn out of this in actuality is for the body to go through the maneuvers; this concrete action can then act with the concreteness of the knowledge of fire burning and bring about an accommodation of the points of dissimilarity. When the Balinese child is chosen (blest or given power), she gets up engrossed totally in imitating her models. Every part of the body must be coordinated in the intricate and sophisticated gestures, and these are the points of concentration. The dance is the function; the structuring of a reverse flow concerning the fire is incidental. (In recent years, this part of the dance is apparently no longer observed.) Generally, the fire was the one used for the preparation of the feast. Dancing through it was simply play. After the play, she returned to the point from which the operation of mind began, the ordinary world in which the fire burns. The little girl knew that she might get some of the festive food roasting beneath the coals and that she would have to be careful to avoid singeing her fingers.

At this point, our Western logic breaks down before an irresolvable paradox. To us, you cannot have it both ways. You cannot dance on the coals without even a blister while beneath those coals pigs and pineapple or whatever are roasting. Frozen in our no-man's-land of confusion between world and reality, having lost the best of both worlds, the organization and the extent of our logic is either-or. Between the either and the or lies a rigorously excluded middle that we Westerners feel we must maintain, else our whole semantic universe will collapse into chaos (as, in fact, it might). And through that excluded middle, ignorant of our logical niceties, the little Balinese child blithely dances.

There are different ways by which the brain can operate on its data and change those data. The Balinese child simply imitates, and any reversing of ordinary cause and effect takes place peripherally and in true play. The father and son stopping the blood and healing the wound did not reverse a process so much as directly operate on concrete material (which is the subject of Chapter 17). Left to his own devices, the child would have bled to death. What they did was through verbal suggestion, the temporary power of the father, and their combined interaction. On their own, the severed artery must bleed, the heart must pump, the fire must burn. They are the world's principles, subject to law, understandable by analysis, standardized and predictable. They constitute the reality of the world or, we might say, physical reality. But add *idea* or abstraction, and you add mind-brain. Add mind-brain to the world, and you have, not reality as it is in the world, but reality as a construction, a created reality. Human reality experience and the world as it is are not synonymous phenomena, although they partake of the same substance. This is why the laws of one operation cannot possibly fit the other, why ordinary scientific testing, which is designed to discover the world's principles, is not appropriate for a study of earth *plus* mind.

Fire walking, the most common of all nonordinary phenomena, takes place all over the world: Greece, Africa, South America, the southeast islands, and almost everywhere in Asia.⁴ (Recently, standard Ceylonese-type fire walking has been done in Canada; a friend of mine, a university professor, took part in one a couple of years ago.) Some of the walking is intense and serious, as in the case of the yearly rituals of the Ceylonese, in which they prepare for the venture with three months of partial fasting, abstinence, and prayer. The firebed they walk (when all are seized) is a deep pit twenty feet across. The heat will melt aluminum on contact. A small percentage fail each year (their faith snaps). Some of these are seriously crippled; others are burned to death on the spot. The majority know ecstacy, the joy of survival, of life over death. They dig their feet into the coals, scoop up handfuls and heap them on their shoulders and heads. Their hair never burns, nor do their garments. They revel in personal power bestowed by the gods.

This personal power consists of a full-dimensional knowledge of the world and its principles, the muscular-mindedness to accept the stress of an unknown-unpredictable, and the logic necessary for abstracting out of concreteness, assimilating and accommodating, and so operating on that information and changing it. All the work of reconstruction goes on beneath the level of awareness. The person is asked only to respond; the conceptual system does the rest.

I am continually asked by those caught in the Western no-man's-land of misplaced concreteness: "But what kind of chemical-molecular changes could the body put forth to alter the effects of fire on flesh?" They are asking for an explanation of the reality created by world plus mind in terms of the limited principles of the world alone. The minute we add mind to the world we get reality experience. Then our neat either-or logical analysis, which may work well with the world itself, no longer works. If a scientist mixed two chemicals in his beaker and got a certain predictable result, he would not likely then insist that he should get the same result from only one of the chemicals. Yet, our academic community does this continually with world and reality experience. Mind is the catalyst that changes the earth into created reality experience, precisely what the earth has moved toward in its 3 billion years of genetic experimentation. Separating mind from world is a massive denial that splits our conscious awareness from our primary process. From his/her split state, the scientist (and fellow victims) rightly concludes that any two-way exchange between earth and human cannot exist; nothing in that split awareness can act back on the hologram in such a manner.

No summation of the unity of the earth as itself can give the infinite flexibility and possibility of world plus mind. The crippling insistence that the earth must on her own display the components of reality experience arises from anxiety. The anxiety arises from our having never had the earth as our matrix. An intelligence whose earth has never formed as matrix can never find a safe place to stand. When the shift of matrix from mother to earth fails to take place, logic has no way to organize concrete patterns into abstractions. We spend most of our lives trying to learn some abstract patterns that our logic can organize. Our young people are beginning to show serious deficits in even this shallow form of abstraction, and we have attributed this to not starting them early enough in abstract thinking itself. But the diametric opposite is the case. We have failed to provide sufficient, mature concrete matrices from which abstraction can truly arise.

All the earth can do with fire is burn, as it is supposed to do. There is no chemical change in the fire or in the child when she walks that fire. There are no molecular shifts, no mind over matter, no mystical mumbo jumbo, no deep esoteric secrets of cosmic space, no hidden pyramid numbers or astrological trickery, no superpowers of flying saucer superminds. The relationship between concept sets and functions in the mind-brain changes, and the relations between mind and its matrix, between microcosmic and macrocosmic hologram, changes accordingly. The functional changes do not take place in awareness; they furnish awareness.

Surely the child has no notion of how her reality experience of fire not burning unfolds for her other than that if *she* does, it does. No more does any of us really know how it is that when we open our eyes, we see the world out there. The structure follows our function of opening our eyes. If the Balinese child did not respond with her single, nonambiguous "yes" to her intent by getting up and doing, if instead she asked our either-or kind of questions, the fire would not have had mind added to its equation and so would simply burn. When understanding structure precedes function, both function and understanding suffer, just as when work is thought to be necessary and play is thought to be something peripheral, the system bogs down. Through the function of play, the work takes place, and creativity unfolds. The missing link of earlier child play is added to the abilities within that child at seven; she walks the fire in play, still responding only to intent, as she did in her first hour. But what accommodates to what? The fire or the flesh? Ah—that is admittedly mystery, thank God, mystery that keeps play and work neatly divided, although they must merge for creation. This is the paradox and the reason that play is the only way the highest intelligence of humankind can unfold.

Chapter 17

The Two-Way Flow:
Assimilation-Accommodation

Uri Geller, for those readers who did not follow this minor-major comedy, was an Israeli entertainer who could apparently bend metal without touching it, make broken or stopped watches run for short periods, and occasionally make an object disappear and who displayed undeniable extrasensory perception. Interested researchers tested Geller's abilities at the Stanford Research Institute in California. The tests were conducted by only one of the dozens of nearly autonomous departments making up this complex (3,000 employees), but those connected with the investigations, which went on for months, were convinced that the *Geller effect* was genuine. Papers stating this opinion were published, and a storm of protest broke out, for academic dogma was brought into question.

So Geller's discrediting was undertaken. Soon we Americans found out, to the disappointment of some and the relief of others that Geller was a fraud, a charlatan, and a cheat. *Time* said so. *Psychology Today* said so. For after all, the Amazing Randy, a professional magician, said so. Andrew Weil, who writes on natural and stoned minds and is an authority, said so. The Amazing Randy, after all, told Andy. And when *Psychology Today* published at length Andy's lengthy report on Randy's exposé, the circle closed. The evidence was in, and Geller was clearly guilty. The Stanford scientists who had been "duped" all those months grew silent, and Geller left the scene.

Then a funny thing happened. Geller went to England in late 1973 to perform his fork-bending stunts on television for the British Broadcasting Company. Geller had observed that people in his audiences occasionally had keys bend in their pockets, rings twist and break on their fingers, and so on while he was doing similar things on the stage. The notion grew that perhaps Geller could operate through people and maybe even at long distance. Or perhaps other people might possess the same odd ability he did. On the English television show, Geller invited all those people out there in television land to join him, to participate in his metal bending by holding forks or spoons themselves to see if the phenomenon might be repeated. Some 1,500 reports flooded the BBC, claiming that forks, spoons, anything handy had indeed bent, broken, moved about—there, in the homes of Britain.

Surely such hysterical claims are often noted, and no validity can be granted such business at all. The funny thing was, the vast majority of the claimants were between the ages of seven and fourteen, the period of suggestibility and concrete operational thinking. The exceptions were a few women, many of whom were not actually holding utensils but found broken, bent, and twisted spoons and such after the show.

When Geller appeared in Scandinavia, Germany, South Africa, and Japan, there were repeat performances. Spoon bending became a popular epidemic. The age bracket ran from seven to fourteen fairly consistently, and the average age was nine.

Had this outbreak occurred in the United States, our analytical psychologists out to defend the strange fantasies of Freud, the brass-tacks realists, the Skinner-box behaviorists would have written learnedly about the deep anxiety syndromes operating to produce such illusions. Agreeing sagely with one another, they would have explained it all away. In England, Germany, Scandinavia, South Africa, and Japan, the reaction was different. At the University of London, for instance, the physics department (headed by John Halstead and under the direct supervision of mathematician-physicist John Taylor) made a genuine scientific response. Just as Aristotle decided to test the common knowledge that salamanders could live in fire by tossing an actual salamander into the fire (whereupon the poor salamander fried to a crisp), so these English scientists tossed some reported Geller salamanders into the fire. They brought a number of the children into the laboratory and began working with them.

Following a slow period in which little happened, the children really began to catch fire. In that encouraging and patient atmosphere, fork bending in many guises began to assert itself. In effect, each laboratory experiment proved another strong suggestion. Each success contributed to the set of expectancy that was beginning to generate. Success breeds success.

During the same period, and operating within his own circuit, Mathew Manning, an English teen-ager, had been doing Geller-type acts since experiencing a poltergeist seizure at eleven years of age. Dr. Brian Josephson, of the prestigious Cavendish Laboratories at Cambridge University (where DNA's double helix was born), winner of the 1973 Nobel Prize in physics and a principal in the investigation of young Manning, said:

> A redefinition of Reality and Nonreality is needed now. . . . We are on the verge of discoveries which may be extremely important for physics. We are dealing here with a new kind of energy. This force must be subject to laws. I believe ordinary methods of scientific investigation will tell us much more about psychic phenomena. They are mysterious, but they are no more mysterious than a lot of things in physics already. In times past, "respectable" scientists would have nothing to do with psychical phenomena; many of them still won't. I think that the "respectable" scientists may find they have missed the boat.

Whether or not Geller was a fraud, then, is beside the point. We have stumbled on a potential that eclipses the investments and institutions of our culture. The full extent of the power of suggestion has just barely been touched upon. Creative logic has been glimpsed. A new aspect of concrete operational thinking has opened. The key to a logic of survival has opened into plain view.

Knowing the intricacies and skill, the long training and hard work necessary to get "the hand quicker than the eye," a legitimate stage magician would never have conceived of asking someone just to imitate him without going through the arduous training. Can you imagine the great Arthur Rubenstein, before one of his uncanny concerts, even conceiving of the notion of inviting his audience to bring along their Steinway or Baldwin grand pianos and, just by listening and watching him, play as he played? Yet this is what Geller did. Surely he gave many hints of extreme naïveté, such as accepting, then aiding and abetting the ridiculous suggestions pumped into him by friends that flying saucer people were responsible for his effects. Surely Geller added to all this and helped build a nonsensical myth that made one cringe with embarrassment. But one reason he proved so gullible was that he had absolutely no idea how his genuine nonordinary phenomena happened and very little control over whether they happened or not. (I qualify his acts by saying "genuine" because it may be that he had low periods during which he padded natural phenomena with plain trickery, but this is beside the point.)

Examine the sequence: An outrageous and impossible suggestion was given over a television network reaching approximately 30 million people, including children of the critical age bracket for being highly susceptible to suggestion. The given suggestion fell squarely into the category of concrete operational thinking in its most tangible form, and the suggestion itself fell into the category of need appropriate to the intent of this period.

Television, the medium through which the children received this suggestion, was (is) the most powerful influence of their lives, every bit as powerful to them as the Balinese rituals in that culture. Television has largely supplanted not only parents as models for imitation but also the child's ordinary fantasy-play projections. Furthermore, television has entered into the structuring of the child's primary world view; indeed, it may be the principal structuring element. Although the resulting shallow, two-dimensional world view ordinarily cripples the emerging primary world view, in the Geller case, with his modeling directly before the children, this tool of enculturation backfired. Happy accident.

No one involved in Geller effects has the slightest idea how the phenomena occur, no more than the Ceylonese understand how they walk fire. Geller effects take place without a person's doing anything and often without a person's even "willing" anything to happen. Concrete operational forms of reversibility thinking are not necessarily conscious or controllable. We can function that way, but we cannot analyze the structure by which such reality experience takes place.

Concrete operations are another stage-specific unfolding of abilities that must be nurtured in order to be activated and developed. Given the suggestion through the most powerful medium for suggestion in their lives, the so-called Geller children saw and did likewise, just as the Balinese child did and for much the same reason. They were imitating, just as they had done in imitative play for years.

The nine-year-old is open to suggestion. S/he has the necessary logic to create the abstract concept involved; s/he has the ability to entertain any state in a continuum of possible states as equally valid; and s/he can operate on concrete information according to suggestions *for* such operation (if s/he is ever lucky enough to receive any). The nine-year-old's world view has not completely hardened. His/her capacities will remain somewhat open until adolescence. In this plastic stage, s/he can certainly accept the idea that a fork can just as easily be a bent, broken, twisted, or altered fork if s/he sees it done. That is immediately an idea for his/her "entertainment." The suggested pattern can easily be extracted from the given pattern in the brain according to the nature of the suggestion. The operation can easily find a sufficient number of points of similarity. The related information from the source of stimulus, that fork itself, is then operated on by this newly created (and arbitrary) pattern, changing that information.

The fact that the source of the sensory stimulus, the fork, changes in this Geller effect introduces new considerations. When the abstract idea operates on the incoming information, the operation changes not only the information but also the source of information. The Balinese child's ability to walk on coals can be attributed to subjective reactions, whatever that might mean. We can see how the body might be so influenced that it does not register pain in the usual way and somehow is not injured as a result. We have heard of Eastern fakirs lying on beds of nails and so on. Research into pain has changed some of our assumptions.

On the other hand, the Geller children are not being subjective. Objects change. The material substance of the world matrix gets altered, and at times, the object just disappears outright. This is what has equally altered the sure academic attitudes of Josephson, Taylor, and many others. There is no return to the state from which this operation of mind begins. That possible state has altered the original. Fire walking is one order of phenomena; causing a metal rod sealed inside a glass tube to tie itself in knots is another. (The Geller children have done a great deal of this.) Both are examples of concrete operational thinking in which the child's logic operates on reality information and changes that information.

In the imitative play of childhood, the child mirrors with his body the body movements of the model. The world is not assimilated to this accommodation. A one-way effect is played on; it in no way affects either child or world, except to give the child a desired play reality and furnish his conceptual machinery its nutrients for world structuring. In fire walking, creative logic may reverse things; the world may assimilate and accommodate to the model, the child. When the operation of mind is over, the basic set of world concepts is there, functioning as it always has and always will. Nothing has changed. The fire certainly does not change; among a group walking it, some may be burned, others not. The world concepts accommodate to the personal act, and the reality of world plus person has been correspondingly changed as needed in that moment and context. This is what the division of labor in the mind-brain system is designed to do. Both processes, earth as itself and person as individual expression, function smoothly within the mind-brain system in an easy symbiotic relation. Thus, the earth achieves her goal of moving beyond her own limitations.

An eleven-year-old Japanese, Jun Sekiguchi, bent a spoon suspended by wire in a sealed plastic container, by "willing it to bend." He made a spoon in the bottom of a basin of water bend without touching it. He threw a spoon into the air, at which point it twisted into a spiral shape. He threw pieces of straight wire into the air, and as they fell, they twisted to form the name of the man running the experiment. None of this was premeditated; it was all random play on the part of the boy. (Only the adult experimenters are so deadly serious; the children find it all hilarious, beaming, smirking, laughing, delighted at each success—and a bit bewildered.)

English children investigated by John Taylor bent metal by stroking it gently with one finger. A twelve-year-old girl made a 40-degree bend in a chrome-plated steel bar by stroking it. An identical bar required 500 pounds of mechanical pressure to bend it in similar fashion. The metal strips that double up into odd shapes inside sealed glass tubes are not touched; the children simply run their hands over the tubes. (Metal is the usual medium for experiment because wood or plastic items tend to disintegrate or explode.)

When Geller visited John Taylor's laboratory in London in June 1974, Taylor had prepared some carefully designed experiments. One involved a pressure-measuring device costing some $600 to construct. The test involved having Geller simply hold the device as the experiment proceeded. As soon as Geller took the device, however, its interior crumbled. Although Taylor quickly seized it, the central diaphragm had disintegrated within about ten seconds. The investment was soon in ruins, and the experiment was a failure. During the same morning, several pieces of copper plate disappeared, only to reappear in other areas of the building. Two of the objects struck Taylor on the back of the leg as he and Geller walked down the hall some seventy feet from where Taylor had last placed them.

These latter episodes fall into the category of poltergeist, or playful spirit, phenomena reported through the ages. Such phenomena have traditionally broken out around early adolescence, just at the period when suggestibility and concrete operations begin to phase out to the stage-specific learnings of adolescence when such abilities atrophy and disappear if they have gone undeveloped. From age seven to about age fourteen or fifteen is the period the biological plan prepares for this learning and development. Uri Geller reports his first phenomena of this sort occurred when he was seven. The phenomena broke into Mathew Manning's life at age eleven. The reason for this random pattern of appearance is hard to determine. The reason why enculturation is more or less effective in varying degrees is hard to say. Research shows that all known psychics received accidental electric shock in childhood, but this is inconclusive. In ordinary successful enculturation, anxiety conditioning systematically screens out each of the bondings and abilities involved as they appear.

In concrete operations, we are dealing with the relation between a primary process and the individual selective consciousness. The primary process encompasses the flow, the world, and the physical body. The young person relates to his/her primary processing in the same way the child relates to his/her mother as s/he builds a knowledge of the world. When the preadolescent's relation with the earth matrix remains in natural balance, a dynamic interaction exists automatically and nonconsciously. To initiate an active, conscious, and selective relation, however, the child must be given his/her initial suggestions for the possibilities. His/her intent still must be given its content from without in order to be brought from potential to actuality. Once the child learns to activate his/her creative relations, s/he can determine some line of action that then gives the cue around which his/her primary process and creative logic can organize. An abstract possibility (one coming, not from the world, but from the mind) can then be extracted out of the given world concepts, and a new reality experience can be created.

Surely all biological organisms exist by interaction between organism and earth, and there is no way to separate the earth from its life. Earth is the planet that lives, that has a twenty-seven-day cycle of temperature change, that has a circulation system for its water, that breathes, that constructs radiation belts to protect its life, that thinks, as Teilhard de Chardin claimed. Seawater cannot be duplicated in a laboratory because it is not just water and salt or this or that but rather a living ecosystem in which the millions of different organisms are all part of the living substance. Separate its life from its water, and you no longer have seawater, that assimilation-accommodation between earth and creature. The lowly slime mold forms a colony on the forest floor that changes the chemical nature of the ground beneath and the atmosphere immediately above. The colony creates a unique environment, a life envelope in which assimilation and accommodation are made by both earth and mold. The mold exists by the grace of the earth's accommodation, just as the earth is a living earth because of creatures such as the slime mold. As you move up the life scale, you move up a scale of complexity of assimilation-accommodation. The earth is always accommodating to the organisms she assimilates and that must assimilate and accommodate to her. No dividing line exists between earth and creature. Remove the creature and earth is a dead rock.

With the human being, the earth's most complex organism, this interaction is as extended and complex as the thought process involved. In fire walking, we have accommodation to the creature through the principles by which the earth operates. In the Geller effect, when metal is transformed without the usual cause-effect mechanisms, some particular object of the earth is assimilated to an idea, and that object accommodates to that idea. There is no break in the continuity and logical flow of the entire life process from seawater, slime mold, chimpanzee, to Geller child bending a spoon by thinking. All we are dealing with is assimilation-accommodation among parts of a living hologram. With the division of labor in the mind-brain system, the possibilities for interaction of such an infinitely complex system become open-ended. That the earth, functioning through and as the child's primary process, should accommodate to her most complex creature according to the nature of that creature's structure is logical and rational.

Yet, precisely at this point of the reversibility of the ordinary flow of assimilation-accommodation, the academic stronghold rises to reject the phenomena. The entire history of Western man rests on the unquestioned assumption that the mind-brain is a *one-way* receptor of information from its world, designed only to interpret and react in adaptive ways to this information. And the only adaptive ways academically recognized and allowed are those using mechanical devices or ineffectual muscular defense stances. This institutionalized belief that the mind has absolutely no influence over or relation to its world except through dominating tools has now created a nuclear terror reducing everyone to total impotence and fate. We deny our true nature at our peril because such denial always creates a demonic counterenergy of destruction. The crux of our social stance is entirely and squarely this issue of our relation of our mind and our reality, our world and our created experience.

At age seven, with his/her world structure largely roughed in and his/her concrete matrix established, the child's system moves toward abstractions on that concreteness and will become organized around whatever suggestions for such abstractions s/he is offered and can assimilate. The flow of interaction between child and matrix is the relation among concept sets or ways for processing information. Abstract concepts can be created in the brain just as they can be drawn out of concrete concepts. Then these patterns can extract accordingly and synthesize experiences outside the world as it is. Abstractions can play on the principles and natural laws of cause and effect as needed. Ordinary effects of the world can be suspended according to the needs and well-being of the particular person, in that person's immediate life envelope. Then the person can operate on and change his context if needed, walk on a bed of fire and not be burned or alter the shape of a potential harm. When the synthetic concepts of operational thinking complete their activity and the world view resumes its concrete activity, a stress-relaxation cycle has been completed. The child's muscular-mindedness to enter into stress-relaxation of this type leads to autonomy. S/he learns that the world matrix meets him/her halfway and augments his/her energy with its own.

Dr. Joel Whitton of Toronto found in his work with Mathew Manning that the old brain (cerebellum and brainstem) seemed to be involved in the actual psychokinesis displayed by Manning. Whitton writes that "psychic functions are not a higher or different degree of concentration . . . but an unknown or outside force that creates it." Because of the involvement of older-brain parts, Whitton suggests that psychic functions are, not random gifts or space-age abilities, but "an innate function and ability in homo sapiens that probably goes back to the earliest history of man."[1]

Perhaps our myths are correct, and our problem is one, not of evolving a higher mentality, but of reclaiming our lost state. Whitton's comment is of interest to me because I have suggested, in my earlier book *The Crack in the Cosmic Egg,* that nonordinary phenomena and primary perceptions would be found to center in older-brain functions. Right-left hemispheric activity cannot account for our most creative interplays. Some of our greatest acts lie, not in brain computing alone, but in interaction with the total life system. Although all the brain systems are involved in any activity, the nature of the activity determines which brain function dominates. The older-brain system, preprogrammed by our genetic plan from the beginning, apparently gives us our creative interactions with the living earth and so is one of our greatest avenues of expression.

Pause with me, then, to consider these 3 billion years of genetic experimenting leading to the human being: moving from concreteness toward abstraction, through thousands of experimental species, to achieve a logic that can conceptualize with unlimited flexibility, an intelligence that can move through infinite realms of content (the more it knows the more it can know), and a means of survival beyond species survival, a personal survival needed by the kind of individual resulting from the development of such an intelligence.

Have these aeons of effort, passing all notions of time as we use the word, had as the goal of this greatest expression magical parlor tricks? Bending spoons? Every movement, every random effect in development has purpose and design. What, then, is the purpose of altering the principles and/or parts of the world itself? These capacities are the logical extension of play, and play is in the service of survival.

Survival play is not developed, of course, and a phenomenon occurs in the children of all cultures somewhere between eight and ten years of age, right in the middle of this concrete stage, a phenomenon that shatters the young life yet receives scant attention. Quietly forming below awareness is a conceptual structure that surfaces as an exquisitely silent anguish, hidden beyond discussion or clarification: the awareness that one must die. The concept of death as one's personal destiny, with no possibility of evasion, unfolds as a function somewhere around age nine. Concepts structure information into meaning regardless of the nature of the concept, and this concept changes everything. Once filtered through this particular abstraction, experience is never again the same. Play disappears and becomes intentional and competitive. The self tries to take over the conceptual work beneath, and childhood dies.

Chapter 18

Toward Autonomy:
Splitting the Brain

Every move that follows intent is adaptive, even that waste of time called play. Development moves toward autonomy, the intelligence to survive. This ability unfolds and operates on two levels: the nonconscious conceptual work within the hologram brain and the conscious self playing on the surface of it. The ability to play on the surface depends on the success of the work beneath, which depends on the success of the play. When play on the surface is finally destroyed and work on the surface becomes the aware self's drive, the inner work of intelligence breaks down, and the synergy of the system collapses. Anxiety takes over, joy disappears, and the avoidance of death becomes the central issue of life. That is, we grow up.

Just as most children learn to walk and get that out of the way before learning to talk, the biological plan strives to get physical learning accomplished and out of the way so that more abstract learning might take place. And in the economy of nature, physical learning provides the transition kinds of concrete abstractions needed to move into full abstract thinking. The physical learning nature expects from the child of seven to about eleven is the art of physical survival, moving his/her body successfully through the tangible living world. Success in physical learning means a complete-enough competence to allow the automatic controls of the old-brain system to take over, freeing intelligence for more abstract matters. Complete physical competence involves not just muscular competence and body prowess but intellectual competence in handling concrete operational thinking. Only through both can physical well-being and security in the world be assured. And until these critical items are assured, intelligence cannot turn such functions over to more automatic controls. Then these late-childhood concerns become the lifelong concerns of an intelligence designed for far greater maturities; all possibilities for abstraction tend to be used for this most concrete and immature need. Intelligence tries to cope with survival while also trying to move ahead with the biological programming and respond to the inner intent for development.

Somewhere around age nine, the biological plan provides that the child should begin to assume responsibility for his/her own survival. By then, s/he should have had two years of modeling and training in the uses of concrete operational thought for survival, as well as the general education of the body. The tragedy is that we learn nothing about survival during this critical period. Instead, we learn a concept of death as practiced and perpetuated by our culture.

Failure to develop the intellectual tools for survival leads to anxiety, just as failure to bond with the mother matrix leads to anxiety in infancy and childhood. Autonomy unfolds out of the logic of differentiation and gives an awareness of separation and independence whether or not any ability to deal with that independence has developed. When unprepared for, independence is sensed by the child as isolation and abandonment. Just as the conditionally bonded four-year-old will have nightmares when individuation begins, the unprepared self feels anxiety at the final functional separations from primary processing, or earth matrix. At this point, it is nature's design to bond and give creative relationship and freedom; but for the unprepared self, the harsh bonds with anxiety deepen.

Just when its brain has been prepared for new learning and cued to look for models to develop physical survival, the child is exposed to the cultural concept of death. This concept is an idea system concerning survival in general: physical, species, and personal. It is an abstraction drawn from abstractions, an idea system growing out of other idea systems going back into prehistory. The idea system has no relation to reality other than the semantic reality it creates, and it offers no techniques at all for actual survival on any level. In fact, the concept of death is a fabric woven of our historical anxiety over having no true technique for survival. History may have begun, such a short time back, when we lost our capacity for survival, and it has been nothing less than the account of the tragedy then befalling us.

Because we fail to develop our genetically given tools for survival, we develop anxiety systems of ideas for possible survival instead. The culture's body of knowledge then arises as the ongoing outgrowth of the concept of death. This body of knowledge is the only thing offered the child as any model for survival; it holds the hopes or pseudo-promises that tools for survival may somehow emerge by serving the idea systems making up that body of knowledge.

In nearly all cultures, the child makes some sort of transition from parent to culture at around age seven. Cultural training in the body of knowledge then begins in order to do two things: First, it moves to break up the natural bonding to the world scheduled to unfold and fully cement at this period and enforces, instead, a bonding to culture. That is, the body of knowledge, with its institutions and priesthoods, becomes the surrogate matrix, presented to the child as the only safe space and source of strength and possibility, which, of course, the living earth alone actually is. Second, this cultural bonding interprets training as instruction in the use of the tools of that culture, both the physical tools of its technology and the mental tools for learning its body of knowledge necessary for developing those mechanical tools.

A concept of death and actual survival ability have no more in common than society and culture have. Failure to develop survival learning leads to the adoption of a concept of death, just as the failure to maintain society breeds the legal system of culture; and, of course, the two go hand in glove. The concept of death conditions one to believe that the greatest chance of forestalling or avoiding death is through success within the institutions that promise death avoidance. One's life image is then locked into sustaining and perpetuating that chosen institution, which can be sustained only by blocking the natural capacity for survival and by maintaining anxiety.

To the prelogical child, death is as different from death to adult logic as the child's play reality is different from the adult work reality.[1] No adult logic concerning the death of the body has meaning to the prelogical child. That child is as yet undifferentiated from the primary process. Such an egocentric self cannot die in the same sense that the grown and isolated self does. An awareness that is not yet articulated from the general awareness cannot comprehend the subject-object split that makes an individual death. Death means disappearance to the child; that which was here is gone. Adult descriptions of why a death took place, what the death means, or even how the death took place will be lost on the child. Such descriptions come only from adult idea systems, all of which are abstractions, having at best only some tenuous threads to the child's immediate concreteness.

The child may agree with and even echo the mouthings of adult logic because s/he is geared to follow cues (and children catch the drift of adult dramatics without grasping the logic). But to think that this agreement means understanding is an error. Few researchers have been able to get around the block of their own logic and find out what a child says about death. Furthermore, adult bias influences the whole set of a child's response. Adult concepts of death are verbal constructions, product of, and subject to, the continual metaphoric mutation within our thinking. In one part of the world, death takes place because of demons; in another, because of ghost enemies (as is the case with a New Guinea tribe that, strangely, has no belief in an afterlife yet is terrified of the ghost of a newly dead person); or because God wills it (dumping the bad on God); or because of demon germs that go bump in the night with our destruction as their evil intent.

The game of peekaboo, which infants love from a very early age, originally meant: alive or dead? That which disappears is dead. Object permanence occurs when the infant's logic retains knowledge that something is still there even when it is not present to the senses. A kind of confused correlation of this is found in the middle-childhood period, when the child grasps death as disappearance and yet does not grasp the irrevocable nature of that disappearance. The child employs a kind of knight's-move logic, shifting ground readily in some makeshift structure.[2] As Rochlin's study showed, when this child is questioned by an adult about death, the question, framed by and within adult logic, and the answer, framed by and within prelogic, indicate mostly the differences of logic and very little about the child's concept of death. "But surely you don't think the dead person still sees?" one researcher asked a five-year-old. The child answered, "No, they can't see, poor things. It's dark in those coffins. But then, at night, when they come outside, they can see then. But not so well."

If a death occurs to one in the child's bond, particularly a parent, that death is interpreted by the child as abandonment. No reason for the abandonment can be given this prereasoning child that can in any way mitigate or explain the disappearance. The dread of abandonment grows whenever the bond with the parents is weak. This dread then becomes attached to his/her ideas about death as disappearance. The dread of abandonment comes from premature autonomy being forced on the child, that is, when the parents make the child aware of, and feel responsible for, his/her own survival. Premature autonomy and survival concerns lead to rapid formation of a concept of death.

Anger is the most destructive force a child knows, and the cultural child develops the idea that a person's death means that someone was angry with that person. Death is also seen as retribution; the person who has died must have done something very bad. The death of a sibling often causes severe guilt because a child often wishes for the death of interfering brother or sister. If the sibling then dies, the child then feels secretly responsible and worries that s/he will be "paid back" (as one child expressed it) or will him/herself be caused to disappear.

The death of a parent is a double-bind guilt to the acculturated child. S/he feels that his/her inevitable death wishes toward the parents for obstructing him/her have suddenly taken effect, and s/he simultaneously undergoes the trauma of abandonment. The child feels that the parent has willfully abandoned him/her, even though s/he also believes that it is his/her fault. The idea of death as permanent and irrevocable is beyond the grasp of this child, whose time is always now, whose place is here, whose world radiates out from him/her, and who is still an integral part of the general flow. Disappearance always has a cause (as in the belief that a parent's death is willfull abandonment), and the child fills in the gaps of his/her logic as best s/he can. His/her prelogic is in no way an evasion by one part of the mind of the real understanding in some other part of his/her awareness. Such studies as Rochlin's interpreting the child's answers as the willfull logic of the child's self-evasion, hiding understanding from conscious awareness, refusing to admit what s/he really knows, are silly and superficial. The child is not hiding from the grim facts when she/he gives such outlandish reasons; s/he is responding as best s/he can to highly loaded and emotionally cued questions. The difference lies, not in truth, but in logical processing of information, including the nature of the adult's question and the child's processing of it.

There are many reasons why death cannot mean to the prelogical child what it means to an adult. The death of a prelogical child is not the same event as the death of a fully individuated person. Physical death and personal death are no more synonymous than world and reality experience. Adult notions of death hinge heavily on being cut off from awareness of the primary process. Furthermore, a concept of death is a construct of verbal logic. The average prelogical child has no capacity for handling high-level verbal abstractions; thus, such a concept cannot begin construction until some ability for abstraction unfolds and is developed. Long before this development, though, the child has absorbed most of the elements of the culture's death concept; it is there, roughed in, ready for the maturation of the necessary logic to act on it and complete it. All the free-floating anxieties of childhood accumulate in a critical mass at about age nine. Then the logical ability unfolds, and the mind-brain makes the ordering of this pattern once it has been given the necessary clues to the nature of that organization.

During the prelogical period, concern over personal survival occurs only when bonding is conditional, incomplete, or broken. The securely bonded child would never conceive of survival concerns; nature provides the child's long dependency precisely so that the parents will assume responsibility for his/her survival and leave the child's system open and free for exploration and construction. Nature provides that the child should not become aware of his/her own survival needs—that is, of death as personal—until s/he has the tools for survival.

Nor does nature mock her children. In the millennia of history, a considerable percentage of children may have died within the first five years of life through natural selection, the gaining of immunities, and general adaptations; but to program a full, conscious knowledge of one's own death into the early years, before any possible techniques of survival could be developed, would be cruel, unnecessary, and stupid.

The magical child's awareness of death unfolds in late childhood in the form of the child's driving desire for autonomy, an awareness of being responsible for his/her own survival. If the child has been given the proper education in survival, this expresses itself as designed: a period of intensive and ecstatic play in which varying the possibilities of one's survival tools are explored, in which concrete operational thinking and enhancement of primary perceptions are practiced. This would mean confrontation, the child actively seeking tests of his/her prowess.

Is this the education he receives? Of course not. At this most critical time, we slap the child into the anxiety-ridden and frightful experience of schooling. For the newly born individual system, this is the equivalent of a violent birth, and the results are pretty much a repetition of that earlier trauma: brain damage, shock, intellectual crippling, and an overall depression that becomes permanent. The great promise with which the child was born is now shattered completely. Each generation produced under schooling proves more shocked, crippled, violent, aggressive, hostile, confused, defiant, despairing, and the social body crumbles faster and faster. And increasingly, our reflexive, conditioned answer is to inflict the tragedy on the child sooner and sooner, in the hope that if we catch him/her early enough, it will all work out. Should we as a species survive our current destructive course, this period of history will be looked upon as a time of delusion and madness far eclipsing that blackest period of the Dark Ages.

The child is doubly caught because schooling has at its roots anxiety over survival, and this web of anxiety is all that is offered the child for modeling at this critical period of survival drive. The child must attend the culture's body of knowledge. If s/he cannot grasp its content and win applause, s/he will still grasp its intention and lose to anxiety. Because what is offered is proclaimed true by parents and superiors, and because there is a system of reward and punishment for success or failure in it, the child has no choice except fall in line. To refuse is to face abandonment by parents and society at large, to have no place left to turn to.

Conceptual structuring takes place below the level of awareness according to the experience furnishing the content. No human would ever willfully construct a concept of death or willfully inflict it on another because this concept presents the entire universe, the life system itself, the world and nature as the enemy. The primary process, one of the three principle functions of the brain system, becomes the dread adversary to be outwitted, avoided, predicted, and controlled by that pitifully inadequate and anxiety-ridden social self. The death concept represents the greater part of the child's own self as the antagonist. His/her newly functional, impressionable, and vulnerable self system is taught to believe that the matrix itself is the enemy. Even the physical body is depicted as that which must be dominated, outwitted, predicted, and controlled if the individual self is to survive. The division of labor has presented a new personality to the world only to have that world represented by adult caretakers as hostile and violent—as indeed it then is as a result of the culture's practice. Then the limited either-or logic of analysis is held to be the only reliable tool available to the child for surviving the adversary world. Life is represented to us as our death, and our analytic brain, only able to pull things apart, is represented as our life.

Examine the roots of every cultural institution and profession: medicine, the military, politics, advertising, television, schooling, life insurance (surely the strangest euphemism ever coined), lawyers, police, news media, weather forecasters, technology as a whole. At the root of any cultural subsystem lies death—the fear, avoidance, and outwitting of death, death as loss of anxiety-reducing possessions, love, youthful looks, vigor, sex appeal, job, security, health, soul, country, and on and on. Each system survives by first either robbing us of our birthright and then selling it back to us or threatening us and then selling us escape from the threat.

The concept of death is a semantic structure. Studies indicate that the so-called dominant hemisphere of brain, the one running the right hand, is the vehicle for this kind of analytic cause-effect thinking. Historically, only this kind of thinking has been considered *right*. Other types of thinking should be left—strictly alone. Right thinking expresses itself in concrete evaluation. Reacting to a situation of threat is suited to this right-handed thinking, and it expresses itself in overt acts that are susceptible to social judgment. (Some societies actually tied children's left hands behind their backs to assure their adherence to right-handed dominance and thus cultural thought.)

Left-handed thinking relates to the primary process, the flow of things, and expresses itself through unity and bonding to the earth. Cultural priests can neither predict nor control a person who operates from left-handed thinking; left-handed thinking has traditionally been considered the weak, threatening, and feminine (exposing male dominance of culture), which is to say that the left hand has been historically associated with death.[3]

Myth and religion are full of left-right imagery, most of which reverses the cultural representation; that is, the left is the true life, and the right is the "broad way leading to destruction." In Norse mythology, the god Odin found the secret spring of wisdom and poetry and asked the guardian of the spring for a drink. The guardian replied: "The price is your right eye." Jesus said if your right eye offends you, pluck it out; if your right hand offends you, cut it off. He said nothing of the left hand, for it represents the flow, the tao, the father or mother (depending on your culture). The Taoists, with their yin-yang symbol (the black being the feminine, the white masculine), understood the true relationship: Each had the other within; each existed only in balance with the other; each arose out of the other.[4]

The structuring of the concept of death takes place in the child unconsciously as a result of nonconscious cueing toward survival, enforced learning of anxiety idea systems, and premature abstract learning (discussed in Chapter 19). This concept is the only survival means then available, and once formed, it operates on all information about the world. Later, all the inner dialogue going on in the head will generate around this concept and its manifold content because concept always functions as concept, a pattern for putting together information. And because survival is the issue of this concept and the concept represents the flow of life as the enemy, all information coming in is subject to its filtering, and it shapes all information from the world according to potential danger or hostility, the final value.

To the primary process and old-brain functions within the mind-brain system, this verbal construct poses a problem. The primary process in the brain is the hologram of the macrocosm; it cannot function as designed and at the same time filter its own function through a conceptual pattern that represents its unifying, creative actions as the arch-adversary. The death concept represents the unified flow as dangerous and the artificial constructs of the culture's body of knowledge and tool capacity as offering the only safe space. How, then, could bonding with the earth, the matrix of all matrices, possibly take place at age seven? How could there be anything but bonding to culture?

Because the primary process is both the larger part of the child's system and the universal flow of things, a paradox ensues. The only solution, if the organism is to continue functioning, is to prematurely transfer all this kind of semantic logic to the dominant hemisphere (the area specializing in analytic thought and orienting to social relations, whence the concept came) through the division of labor within the brain. Then the subdominant hemisphere and old brain can continue to function according to plan, which means keeping the organism actually alive and functioning on the earth.

So somewhere around nine or ten, language, at least as it is used for propositional logic, becomes the specialty of the dominant hemisphere, along with the volitional decision making of our either-or survival logic (which originates in flight-fight reactions). The combination of these two effects is overpowering. The child's conscious awareness is literally forced to attend to this system of thought, lock in on the promises that the culture holds for manipulation of this semantic logic as a way of avoiding anxiety, and screen out the older life systems as culture demands. In a neat double bind, the primary process and body-knowing are then essentially mute because they do not partake of this analytic language (partly in order to be free of the concepts semantic logic holds). Meanwhile, schooling (acculturation) throws a continually greater emphasis on semantic structures. The word-built world becomes the only harbor for the newly forming independent mind, and social consensus begins to crowd out a criterion of balance within. The result is a neat cleavage, a splitting of the brain without surgery. The self system is pitted against the rest of the brain system; we feel isolated and estranged from our world (the large adversary), from each other (potential adversaries), and even from our own body.

By the time the child is ten or eleven, logic has matured sufficiently to handle the premature abstractions that schooling enforces and the problems of premature autonomy brought about by the death concept. But the stage-specific period for bonding to the earth and the possibilities for operational relations with that earth begins to fade at age eleven and largely disappears around age fourteen or fifteen. The biological plan moves ahead, and the young person is left to struggle on with only the culture's concept of death and its body of knowledge.

After age eleven, as new logical shifts take place, logical development depends on internalizing and abstracting speech.[5] At some point during preadolescence, words should begin to dissociate fully from the objects named so that thinking can begin to stand outside concrete thinking and achieve objectivity. A premature dissociation of name and thing named works against the movement from concrete operational thinking toward a purely abstract form of operational thinking. After the child has reached age eleven, language is *meant* to be separated from the body-knowing kind of concrete language because by then, all concrete learnings should have been perfected and become virtually autonomic. But anxiety conditioning has acted on what should have been a natural division, brought it about prematurely, and created a nearly unbridgeable split rather than a separated but functional relation.

The cultural reality system is based on a word-built logic with only the most tenuous threads of association with the real world. This semantic reality is extremely unstable. It must be carried in the brain system by only a portion of that system. Yet, the young person has no other place to turn. How does the self system try to stabilize its very shaky reality premise built on semantic logic? Through a continual inner play of words, or *roof-brain chatter.*[6] A semantic reality is kept intact through unbroken semantic feedback, but the word-built world receives little support from the real world, which is not a semantic proposition. So the person's awareness system becomes one vast arena for internal word arguments. This starts as primary processes fade and give way to the dominance of anxiety conditioning and cultural semantics.

Autonomy does not develop; it gives way to an awareness of death, conceived by a culture that has not developed a logic of survival, that can never leave the concrete stage that opens at age seven, that develops only its inherited anxiety over having no ability to survive. In such a culture, physical survival and personal survival become as confused as reality experience and the world.

A common theme in the dreams of seven-, eight-, and nine-year-olds is death and resurrection in various forms. A theory of ghosts seems to spring up in these children of its own accord. The child concerned over a death in his/her family will often dream that the person returns to him/her and gives the child his or her life energy. Naturally, we dismiss these dreams as psychological compensations for loss or evasive maneuvers to avoid the awful facts the child does not want to face. That is, if the child's dreams take such a constructive, helpful, and optimistic form, they are put into the same category of wish fulfillment as childhood play. Both are considered techniques for avoiding adjustment or adaptation to the harsh realities of life (at least that is how the priests of the anxiety systems view them). Perhaps, if we took our cues from our children, we would find that their dreams are trying to tell them something, just as their play tries to tell us something. Children often try to tell us what we in our blindness and deafness have so seriously failed to tell them.

Chapter 19

The Cycle of Creative Competence

The parents of the magical child lead him/her into the possibilities of the world by example. At seven, s/he is open to suggestion, able to construct the abstractions needed for moving into the world according to ideas about the world, and able to operate on world information and change that information according to idea. To the child, the parents are playing with him/her, joining in his/her reality. To the parent, the child is playing with them, joining them in ever deeper play with the principles of mind.

The child is fascinated with the world and becomes analytic. S/he wants to take the world apart and see what makes it tick, and s/he will, in the coming years, take apart the clock, a watch, the electric mixer, the sewing machine, or whatever is available. This, too, is learning, and the parents make available things for the youngster to operate on, not just educational toys, but things of the real adult world. They allow the child to bumble through projects, helping only if asked. They have patience when s/he takes apart but cannot reassemble, which is often the case. They know that his/her logic is not yet reversible, that s/he will follow the impulse for taking apart but will have difficulty reversing his/her steps and remembering how to put together again.

Doing things is the order of the child's day; s/he thinks by doing. S/he cannot yet extricate him/herself from body actions and observe them. The parents do not restrain body action in favor of some arbitrary head action appropriate only to later stages, because they know that at this stage body restriction is intellectual restriction.

Through creative modeling, they furnish the youngster with the principles of mind needed for moving beyond the principles of the world. They discuss as matters of fact areas currently explored as biofeedback training. As a matter of course, they lead the child to become aware of his/her body and assume personal power over it. For instance, to expand on the example I gave earlier, the child cuts his wrist seriously; the father responds according to the needs of the situation, picks the child up, reaffirms the bond, and gives the safe space. He holds the injured limb, looks the child in the eye, smiles to establish the calm of control, and invites the child to join him in stopping that blood. To the bonded child, the parents are omnipotent, and their word is truth. At eight, the child is highly suggestible and cued for survival learning. The parents combine verbal suggestion with imitation by asking the child to join them. The child's brain can make such abstractions if they draw on tangible concreteness, such as the body or the immediate world. Through sparse, terse, concrete language, the father instructs the child in energy direction, suggesting that the blood stop flowing. They mirror the idea to each other, entertaining this possibility. They function as though it is occurring, and form follows function; the conceptual work beneath the awareness follows suit.

Just as the Balinese child could, at such a point, walk the fire and not be burned, so this child's brain immediately assimilates the father's instructions and his body accommodates to the operations of mind. The blood loss stops, and the wound begins to heal. (Again, this is not hypothetical. I am simply reporting. I could add examples from personal experience.)

What are the possibilities of suggestion to the concrete operational child? The implications stagger the imagination. We draw back and dismiss the potential; our deeply ingrained pessimism over the human condition forces our surrender to professionalism. I would suggest that you examine current research into biofeedback training to gain a marginal glimpse. Limited facets of body control are heralded as major achievements, as they are indeed for a split system because these applications are attempted years after the stage-specific unfolding of such abilities. The magical child would, of course, pick all this up automatically and playfully, between the seventh and fourteenth years, if given education in such avenues to well-being. The only limits to the possibilities of concrete operational thinking are set by the parents' own belief system, capacity for creative thought, willingness to leave consensus and to assume responsibility for expanding the criteria for the resulting parent-child reality experience.

Professionalism and the institution grow out of our fear over reality criteria. In the case of the injured child, for instance, the average parent would have little capacity for responding to the needs of the situation. S/he would, instead, react. Conditioned to surrender personal power and ability to the professional, the parent would have to rush the child to a hospital or doctor. Even if s/he knew of the personal possibilities for power in such a situation, fear of social condemnation (if s/he failed) would prove incapacitating and would force him/her to react rather than respond.

The child whose parent panics and rushes him/her to the professional (that person who stands between self and personal power) undergoes a deep and abiding learning. S/he learns that the parents do not have the personal power s/he believed them to have. S/he learns that the parents cannot act on his/her behalf, that the matrix is not the safe space, the place of power and possibility, that these must be bought from the professionals. Muscular-mindedness grows by finding that when one gestures to the matrix, the matrix gestures back with a mirroring and enhancing of power and possibility. The parent who panics and shifts responsibility thus dispels the child's own sense of personal power and ability. The child learns that s/he is as impotent as the parents. The stage is then set for the child's own surrender of responsibility to the professional. Later, as a parent, s/he, too, will have no choice but to react in panic and throw him/herself on the mercy of the professional (at their astonishing prices). His/her child's growth and education will, in turn, also be in the lack of the power to act.

The human body is an infinitely complex interaction of creative forces, all achieving a miraculous homeostasis. Seldom does this balance need conscious attention, but when such attention is needed, the body gives clear signals through a well-developed system. Our volitional awareness is then expected to make the necessary adjustments; the decision-making part of the hologram must act back on the more automatic parts. Through acculturation and the surrender of competence to the professional, awareness of the body's language and response to it are lost. Then the professional is the only hope left, and, of course, s/he capitalizes on our incompetence and works to keep us incompetent (lest s/he should have no return business).

So the parents of the magical child educate their youngster in body signals and corresponding responses. An ache or pain is heeded as a fire alarm is. They learn to look for that fire, not to disconnect the bell with drugs. (Physician Irving Oyle likened chemotherapy as now practiced to speeding down the highway, spotting your oil-failure indicator light flashing on, and responding by pulling out a revolver and shooting out that light.)

As the child grows older, the parents use more verbal instruction for concrete operations. Verbal suggestions for concrete operations within the child's body are effective because the child's language is not yet fully separated from its concrete referents. That is, language is not yet fully abstracted. The child of seven to ten or eleven still thinks in actions and acts his/her thinking. Language is still of the body, although the separation of word and thing is under way. The child is now capable of patterning concrete information through such abstractions and so of operating on the information. In no category is this logic more appropriate than body monitoring and emergency control, particularly during preadolescence.

The parents capitalize on the magical child's belief in their omnipotence. They encourage his/her innate idea that they have power in their world and that through them s/he can share in this power and develop his/her own. Should the child become ill for some reason (although for the bonded child, such unwholeness is rare), the parents assure him/her that they have the personal power to heal. They then devote their full attention to that healing because far more than a temporary body misalignment is involved. Learning is involved; the development of the ability to interact is at stake. Through a continual suggestion, reassurance, and reaffirming of their power and their ability to lend him/her that power, the child's suggestibility receives the idea of healing, and the inner work responds. The child learns that mind has dominion over the world.

Throughout this period, the parents have continued to encourage, enhance, and respond to the child's primary perceptions. They practice telepathy by using the hypnagogic and anagogic periods right before sleep and on first waking. During these brief periods, they exercise this capacity with their child just as assiduously as a parent might exercise toilet training. They practice remote viewing, encouraging the child to sense particular target areas chosen for the day and to report his/her sensing to them. Through such play, these primary perceptions grow enormously during the stage of suggestibility because the parents are suggesting and entering into specific experiences with the child.

Learning to transform objects, as exhibited by the Geller effect or walking fire without harm, may have no practical application within ordinary life, but these nonordinary events do far more than just give possibilities for specific concrete acts of protection. They give enormous confidence in personal power, the power of the mind to flow with the principles of the earth and go beyond the limitations of either. This is the great learning within concrete operations. Personal power—the muscular-mindedness to enter into ever more abstract and complex unknown-unpredictable situations—is always the issue.

Of course, intelligence is not limited to bodily concerns. The child has an insatiable curiosity about everything and desires to interact with a wide spectrum of possibilities. He loves to handle logical learnings of a wide sort. Many exercises in intelligence match his intent. Music is eminently suitable from age four on because it is pure body response and action. Its visual symbols are, not abstractions or symbols in any sense, but visual signals for muscular response, a sensorimotor learning. Learning to read music and learning to read words are worlds apart. They have no points of similarity and involve radically different internal processes. Mathematics and logic of a concrete nature are appropriate after age seven. Art, dance, and all body movements are appropriate as long as they remain play. Should some particular study not match his/her intent, the child will not learn that activity because s/he will not be able to play in it. The parents know that enforced attendance indicates inappropriate activities and that an increased ability to interact will not take place. The child is given exactly the same freedom of aesthetic response to intellectual samplings that s/he was given to food samplings. The parents know that the child cannot be artificially motivated to learn; they know that s/he is already motivated by the strongest driving force on earth: his/her inner intent. They know that when they take cues from this intent and respond with an appropriate modeling, the child automatically and unhesitatingly follows.

Little by little, the child's play on the surface and his/her conceptual work beneath the surface move closer to synergy, which will finally unfold during adolescence in full reversibility thinking. This synergy takes place as the child learns to be selective about what s/he selects from the continuum of possibilities to be given fantasy-play reality. His/her use of imagination and fantasy have been free-ranging, as they should have been. Now, with the growing rewards and successes from concrete operations, his/her capacity for imagination becomes more devoted to the needs of physical survival and well-being in this world, and in this way outer and inner increasingly mesh.

The parents know that their child needs solitude and quiet. Just as they avoid exposing the child to sensory overload, they avoid overloading his/her life with demands. S/he needs long stretches of unfilled time, particularly during the last plateau of his/her learning cycle (during the tenth and early eleventh years). S/he needs time for mental staring. Just as s/he stared for long periods during the early stages, creating empty categories of possibility to be filled in with full sensory exploration, s/he now stares conceptually, creating empty categories of thought to be filled in with abstract explorations. Thought for thought's sake is beginning to structure within. Regulatory feedback is feeding back on the abstractions made out of the child's operational interactions with the world. When regulatory feedback extracts out of these initial abstractions drawn from concrete concepts, logic is achieving secondary abstraction. This is thinking about thinking. The brain is beginning to function on its own products and processes and to be less dependent on the world. The logic of differentiation is beginning to separate the thought from the action or event.

The parents know that between seven and nine, their child needs interaction with them and with superiors first and interaction with peers second because intent within must always get its content from without and only parents and superiors can furnish his/her intent with content at this period. Premature peer interaction indicates a failure of parental bonding and earth bonding. A child bonds to his/her peers only as compensation. Peer bonding cannot lead to development until around age ten simply because one child's intent cannot furnish another child's intent with content. Intelligence will not grow this way. Peer interaction should unfold during the practice and variation period of the learning cycle (late in the ninth year and during the tenth) and not much before. Then the structured content of each preadolescent can find consensus and support in the practice and variation of group play.

After age nine, the child's logic of differentiation will begin to separate the word and the thing denoted by that word. Language is moving toward, although it has not become, a separate thought process in the brain. The newborn synchronizes body movement to speech; the two-year-old moves his hand as he says "hand"; the four-year-old coordinates body movements and senses through language. Language is a body movement and acts as a coordinate of the whole system, just as vision does for the senses. The name of a thing enters into the early child's brain pattern for putting information about that thing together, and that name is an integral part of the thing or event, not a description of it or symbol for it. This concreteness of language is a permanent part of the primary process and old-brain body-knowing. That is the reason the eight- or nine-year-old can be given a verbal suggestion for operating on concrete information; in the concrete concepts of his mind-brain, word and thing named are still a unit, and the thing can be changed through the word.

Logical feedback is always separating knowledge into more sophisticated categories through feeding back over experience. When separation of word from thing begins in late childhood, this separation does not affect the concrete concepts of the primary process or body-knowing; they remain inviolate. The abstraction of language involves the division of labor. Thus, the kind of language to be continually refined and synthesized in logic's feedback will grow completely abstract and no longer related to the concrete language of primary process and old brain. The maturing intelligence will then have (or should have) these three distinctly different but functional language uses at his/her disposal: concrete, abstractions from concreteness, and pure abstractions. Intent precedes and prepares for the ability to do. A new logical shift is in store at about age eleven, a move toward pure abstract thinking. Separating the word from what it names is part of this moving toward formal thought. Only then should a word be descriptive of or stand for that object or event. For the higher logical abilities to develop, language must become separated from concreteness and become a self-enclosed system. This refinement should not, however, be bought at the expense of the concrete language of the body or the language of a primary process.

When we force the child to work prematurely with abstract thought, we break up the vital unity of self and world. "Writing," Vigotsky explains, "virtually enforces a remoteness of reference on the language user." Writing (and to a lesser extent reading) enforces a separation between name and thing named. To deal with this kind of abstraction, the logic of differentiation is forced to skip all preliminary steps and prematurely begin such a separation. The result is an enforced separation between self and world, even though the differentiation required is still clumsy and inadequate. (Thus, Furth claims premature literacy stops the development of intelligence cold for two to three years.)

The shift of matrix from earth to self and from self as mind-brain and body to mind-brain alone, as genetically planned, depends upon and demands such a separation between self and world. The separation is the same as that between infant and womb, child and mother, and self system and primary process. The issue is, *when* should self and world functionally differentiate? Nature provides that this separation take place somewhere around age ten or eleven, when concrete operations have been roughed in and become matters of practice. Premature separation, as brought about by premature literacy, creates the equivalent of a premature birth, a wrenching out of context that creates an isolation and abandonment which we then rationalize as "individuality."

Bruner noted that learning to read and write had a huge impact on children in the Belgian Congo, "forcing them to communicate out of the context of their immediate reference." That is, literacy forced the children to separate their sense of self from their actions, thoughts, and world experiences. This is the same phenomenon he observed with the East African Wolof children, whose thought and the object of thought seemed to be one until taught to read and write. This leads to a key statement and the crux of this issue: "School seems to promote the self-consciousness born of a distinction between human processes and physical phenomena." And indeed it does. But is this what we want in the years from seven to eleven, when such premature separation breaks up the functional unity between individual and world system, and limits concrete operational thinking?

The issue rests on biological functions within the brain. The late child's conceptual system consists of patterns of sensory organization formed through his actual sensory interaction during his developmental years. The written word is made of infinitely variable symbol letters that can be arranged in groups to stand for symbols, which stand for words, which must *then* stand for things or events. The actual pattern in the brain includes the word as an integral part of the thing or event, the way by which word can act as a coordinate between mind-brain and body and as a coordinate between brain and earth system. This gestalt must be artificially and arbitrarily broken up for literacy learning at age six or seven.[1] The word portion of the unified conceptual pattern must be wrenched out of context and treated as an isolated entity, and three different levels of abstraction of that concreteness must be performed. Because the brain operates as a unit, this differentiation acts on all the computer brain's concepts, including the self system's sense of awareness in the world system, leading to the sense of alienation, isolation, and psychological abandonment that contribute to formation of the concept of death at around age nine.

When do we want to "promote the self-consciousness born of a distinction between human processes and physical phenomena"? Surely not at age seven or eight, just when the new self is emerging in a functional relationship with the primary process. That innate and intuitive connection is nothing less than our bonding to the earth, which is literally our umbilical cord through which our nourishment and substance must come at this critical stage. The matrix shift at age eleven is the appropriate time for these distinctions. Thus, the parents of the magical child avoid premature or enforced separation of word from thing and the resulting separation of self and world. They delay literacy until age eleven. The child's system maintains its one-for-one correspondence between thing and name in order that s/he might learn to operate on that information when necessary and change it as needed for physical well-being.

Around age nine, with two rich years of operational thinking and some four to five years of continual enhancement of primary perceptions bonding him/her with the earth matrix, the magical child moves toward autonomy. Through logical maturation, s/he becomes aware that his/her body is vulnerable and that the parents' assumption of his/her well-being has limits. S/he longs to assume responsibility for his/her survival. With a background of survival learning and practice and with bondings with the earth, s/he has confidence in his/her own ability to respond to life. His/her response is the excitement of adventure. Just as a person with a new game or skill desires to test that skill under fire, so the magical child desires confrontations with his/her own survival.

Logical maturation brings awareness of death as a possibility in every unfolding moment, but this knowledge adds zest to living. The stress of the unknown-unpredictable is an exciting challenge rather than a source of anxiety and dread. Awareness of death acts as the catalyst on all the child's knowledge, fills in the details of his/her roughed-in survival ability, and brings alertness to his/her acts. Death gives meaning, purpose, and design to his/her survival skills. Child play becomes the deep play of late preadolescence and adolescence, play in which the young person is aware of how high the stakes are and so desires to increase his/her skills and up the ante.

Muscular-mindedness, then, is the ability to accept a knowledge of death without anxiety and so be strengthened, rather than weakened, by it. Surely the child will know fear, and s/he will have been educated to have a healthy respect for that fear. S/he will learn to heed and use fear as ongoing learning because fear is the body's signal for alertness. Fear has an object and gives a point for concentration, a focus for applying survival skills. Anxiety has no concrete object and so cannot organize the system into focus. Anxiety divides the intent against itself and weakens survival ability. The anxiety-ridden system reacts to the unfolding event, trying to use the ability to interact as a buffer between self and some potential harm. Anxiety does not evaluate the situation as the chance to exercise the ability to interact; it screens the actual information from the event through a preset criteria based on reaction.

During preadolescence, the child longs for adventure and excitement. His/her muscular-mindedness for coping with high stress needs exercise, just as any other act does. Peer group or social orientation becomes increasingly appropriate. There is a high accident rate among children between age ten or so and later adolescence (before the age of the automobile). Young people in this age bracket will compulsively take extraordinary risks. The preadolescent is impelled to confront danger, just as s/he was earlier impelled to interact with his/her world with all his/her senses. The tragedy is, of course, that the cultural child is given no tools for this encounter, yet his/her biological plan unfolds the intent on schedule, just as though s/he had been actually educated.

I remember this so well from my own preadolescence: We were driven to risks beyond rhyme or reason. We had a game called *back out,* a form of follow the leader, and the biggest, bravest, most athletic boy, Wendy, was always leader. He would suddenly jump up, shout "back out," and rush off into harrowing feats, with the rest of us flying after him with equal dread and thrill. We dreaded being incapable of keeping up or backing out through fear. Scaling the cliffs at Flag Rock; up the old school building's fire escape to the fourth floor, inching our way around the crumbling cornice; leaping from the peak of the barn; crawling beneath the coal cars jolting about as a train was made up; rushing down through the unknown terrace neighborhood, where homes were built on a steeply pitched hillside, a hedge coming up, the leader hurdling it with a magnificent leap, only to disappear silently. And each of us, unable to break stride or because such a leap was impossible, rushing pell-mell toward that moment, secretly weeping and wetting our britches; the leap up, over, a long fifteen-foot drop onto a steep slant, each tumbling out of the way of the next hurtling, white-faced body; shaken, breath knocked out, gasping, but instantly up and running blindly on. Competitiveness? No. It was our inner drive impelling us into confrontations we did not understand, an intent without content. And then Wendy's great dive, from a limb higher than anyone had ever dared before, into the rock-encircled swimming hole; missing by a mere six inches or so; and our long haul of his body, head lolling strangely, back to town, where help could not help.

We were impelled by our intent to test ourselves, yet had no notion of how to go about it, no understanding of what impelled us or what might be appropriate to our needs. We had to furnish ourselves with peer-constructed content, and our notions of content were crude. Dares, taunts, and cruelties could not substitute for the education that had been sorely neglected. Instead of survival techniques, we had only our culture's anxieties, and our bravado and daring proved poor substitutes against the ironclad principles of a world we did not understand.

In the years from nine to eleven, the period of practicing operations on concrete knowledge, the magical child has a wealth of experience in abstracting out of concreteness. His/her parents assume an increasingly peripheral, supportive role. They know their child must learn autonomy by practicing it. They have equipped him/her with all the techniques for survival available to them and have guided his/her introduction into thinking about thinking. They will have another critical period of modeling and guidance, but they know s/he is rapidly moving toward becoming his/her own matrix. They stand behind him/her with physical support; their bonding is unbroken and unquestioned. By the child's eleventh or twelfth year, however, their job is nearing completion, and they prepare to retire to more invisible supporting roles with grace. Before long, even that support will not be needed. Having had their own greatest learning through being the teachers, the parents are then ready to shift into other modes themselves.

The child's intelligence at eleven is some two-thirds developed. S/he has a knowledge of his/her world; s/he relates creatively with it; and s/he survives within it. S/he has personal power and freedom from anxiety, imagination, and creativity. Yet everything taking place in these first years has been preparatory to the great possibility unfolding in formal operational thinking. This is the journey into the mind, the creation of realities, the point at which the logical structuring beneath the surface merges fully with the play in awareness.

Chapter 20

Thinking about Thinking:
Formal Operations

During World War II, the U.S. army set up air bases in Alaska. Time and again, mechanics reported that they would be frustrated by some engine fault, only to have some ignorant Eskimo handyman amble up, peer over their shoulder, smilingly reach over into the bowels of the engine, tinker with some gadget, and repair the machine.[1] Apparently, this was similar to those so-called idio savants who cannot read or write but can do astonishing mathematical computations in their heads without knowing how. The Eskimo seemed to follow the dictates of his primary processing, allowing his body to move appropriately in much the same way as Ootek sensed the location of the caribou, the direction of the weather, and the natural flow. But his ability to open to primary perceptions and move accordingly with the machine was not then reversible; that is, he could not stand outside his own actions, analyze them, and come to an understanding of the machine or of machinery in general. Uncanny as his talent was, in itself, it would probably never lead to the pure inventiveness to build that machine.

The Balinese child or the Ceylonese who can entertain the possibility of fire not burning as an equally valid state returns to the point from which the operation of mind began. But this is a return in purely concrete terms, a return to the earth matrix as it is. These people cannot retrace their steps, analyze them, and come to an understanding of what their body-knowing has accomplished. Thus, they never learn to take their miraculous ability and apply it freely to other activities.

Somewhere around age eleven, the brain undergoes another growth spurt. At the same time, another logical shift takes place, giving new ways of processing information. Susceptibility to suggestion hits its peak, from which it will slowly phase out as one of the characteristics of the mind-brain by about age fifteen. Formal operational thinking, the ability of the mind to operate on and change information its own brain, unfolds for development. As usual, it is only an intent within and must receive its initial impetus from outside sources, but this dependency on modeling will fade as the new ability develops. The thrust of the biological plan during this period is for the mind-brain to become its own source of possibility.

At age nine, the child could learn a concrete operation by model or instruction, but s/he could not correlate what s/he had learned. By nine, s/he has the ability to operate on his/her incoming information and change it according to an idea s/he has grasped (e.g., discovering that the liquid in a fat, short flask does not become more liquid when poured into a tall, thin flask). Heretofore, tall and thin meant bigger and more in the child's short-statured world. But suddenly, operational thinking grasps the notion of conservation, that the amount of liquid is constant regardless of the shape of the flask it is poured into. S/he will have to go through the same steps of discovery in other problems of conservation, such as being shown a small figure of modeling clay, then rolling the figure out flat, making a very large figure, and being asked which one has the most clay. Until some logical maturation has occurred, s/he will not correlate the discovery of the liquid with the problem of the clay. At some point of logical maturity, s/he reverses his/her steps and realizes more than just a single fact of conservation by realizing the overall law of conservation. S/he can then correlate and apply the principles of one discovery over a wide range of roughly similar problems.[2]

When the child first discovers that the liquid remains constant, s/he has abstracted from the concrete knowledge gained in his/her earlier years. This can be called a *first-level abstraction,* one arising directly out of practical intelligence. It is based on a concrete pattern for putting together actual sensory information. But then, in the further refinement of logic, when the child grasps the principle of conservation and realizes that it applies universally, s/he has grasped, or created in the brain, an abstraction of that first-level abstraction. At that point, thinking is operating on itself. The child is thinking about thinking, whether s/he is aware of it or not. This grasp of the principle involved is a *second-level abstraction.*

During the years from seven to eleven, a body of first-level abstractions should have formed. The variety of appropriate concrete abstractions has been detailed: the logic of concrete logic; arithmetic; operations on the physical body, such as stopping a wound from bleeding or stopping pain; the various Geller effects and cause-effect reversals. All this activity creates a first-level abstract body of knowledge that logical feedback will start feeding back on (once it has been roughed in and becomes functional), synthesizing, and making categories of these preliminary forms of abstraction. By age eleven, with a shift of logic and a brain-growth spurt, logic will be able to create abstractions through this abstract ability itself. The brain then will have a critical mass of first-level abstractions offering a wide continuum of points of similarity for *second-level abstractions,* which are pure ideas that do not have to be related directly to concreteness. This is *formal operational thinking.*

Through formal operations, the mind can experience information and perceptions from its own creative thought alone. Out of its vast pool of knowledge, the brain can then create its own stimuli and experience perceptions from its own abstract conceptions. Thus, suggestibility will eventually be phased out as a needed tool. The magical child's perceptual experience will then have a wide source of possibility: relating to the earth as it is, a matrix of stable background that is experienced every day; creatively relating with that earth through concrete operations of mind, giving possibilities beyond the earth's own principles of cause and effect; relating with the possibilities of pure thinking, imagination, abstract conceptual constructions and the resulting perceptual experience (not found in any concreteness or operation on concreteness), which means a reality created entirely within; and mixtures of these three ways of processing and/or creating information. To this last category must be added the possibilities of one person creating abstract perceptual experience and sharing it with another person or persons and the interactions between them in creating consensus realities.

Formal operations depend on objectivity. For these, you must be able to stand outside yourself and observe your own actions. Thought must be able to separate from what is thought about. This is the objectivity lacking in the East African children until those children were taught to read and write. Separating self from world is one of the prerequisites for separating thought from what is thought about, which in turn depends on separating the word from the object or event named by that word. All this differentiation has been part of regulatory feedback's job in late childhood and early preadolescence and remains its job until the young person reaches fifteen or so.

Nature provides for this gradual detachment so that concrete operations might be learned, perfected, and turned over to more autonomic processes in the old brain as part of the whole substrata of automatic information processing.

Remember that language formed in the infant as bodily movements; that the two-year-old moved his/her hand as s/he said the word; that the four-year-old employed language as a coordinate of bodily movements. The word *hot* formed as a part of the general brain pattern for fire, which also included the physical recoil response when needed. In concrete operations, this word-thing unity still played the major role in the conceptual work of the brain hologram relating with the earth hologram. Through the logic of differentiation, a word begins to be abstracted from this unity and stand alone as a discrete unit of thought. A word then stands for or represents a thing or event. Then thinking inside the head, as opposed to thinking as action, is possible. A logic of words independent of any physical reality can then develop, and this is the propositional language of the adult, another aspect of the formal operations that open around age eleven. That is why literacy is so easily introduced to the eleven-year-old; at this point it does not create premature autonomy and abandonment.

At age eleven, the young mind still needs examples and guidance in order to build a sufficient body of pure abstractions. Suggestibility is at its peak at this period. At age seven, the child's suggestions for possibility needed to be given in concrete form, directly in front of him/her, or by specific concrete instruction and suggestion. His/her capacity for imitative play then moved his/her body accordingly, and the new abstract concepts were formed out of this concrete action. At eleven, suggestions can be given without direct modeling or concrete referent. The eleven-year-old Japanese, Juni, simply heard a newscast about children repeating Geller's exploits. Juni immediately knew he could do so and did. John Taylor found that older children and teen-agers could imitate after only hearing of some possibility; they had a sufficient ability to create abstractions not based on concreteness.

The nature of abstractions given the eleven-year-old must have a sufficient number of points of similarity with his/her existing abstract knowledge to be assimilated and a sufficient number of points of dissimilarity to bring about accommodations and new conceptual ability. Following that brain-growth spurt, the eleven- or twelve-year-old has a passion for learning, a passion for ideas, a universal longing to understand. I remember the long, late-night talks my buddies and I had at that stage, as we slept over at each other's houses or out under the stars, rolled up in old army blankets.

We understood more than adults had any idea of, and we longed to know and comprehend everything. We were filled with long, serious thoughts, engrossed in thinking about thinking. At twelve and thirteen, we ranged over universal issues: the vastness of space and time, the overwhelming problem of God, the meaning of existence. There were few limits to our journeying into thought along whatever skimpy lines opened for us. None of our longings were met by schooling. We found few points of correspondence between our vast hunger and the strange, harsh fare fed us at that board. Somewhere before maturity, however, our anxieties drove us to accept the alien point of view we were schooled in, and our longings were lost in the mad push for identity that filled our next decades, a push that lost us the world and all its offerings.

The parents of the magical child know that the periods of intensive learning ushered in by brain-growth spurts do not last. They are aware of the cycle of competence to be followed at each new stage. New learning is appropriate for about a year and a half after the growth spurt; this is the period of roughing in the new possibilities and capacities. The only additional learning that occurs during the filling-in-the-details period is that which augments and completes the initial learning. And the parents know that in the final third or so of the cycle, when practice and variation are called for, no new learnings are appropriate. During this period, they largely leave their child alone, interceding only as his/her practice and variation need specific help. They know that a slow, steady, progressive accumulation of knowledge, which unfortunately is believed by educators to be possible, is, in fact, not possible and specifically damaging if attempted. They take their cues from their child and respond accordingly.

They know that their child is biologically geared for learning and will do so automatically and joyfully when the content offered meshes with his/her intent and its needs. They know that the child is driven from within to learn and that attempts at exterior motivation can induce only anxiety-conditioned reactions, not learning. They know their child is genetically programmed to be led and guided. They know that the child's play on the surface and conceptual work beneath are moving into closer synchrony, leading toward the point when s/he will be able to play freely with an infinite potential.

The meshing of play and conceptual work is the whole thrust and meaning of development and the way by which we move from concreteness to abstraction. Earlier, we saw how the early child's play remained distinct from the conceptual construction of his/her world view. At age seven, when individuation begins to function, play can, if trained or guided, begin to mesh with concepts, as we noted in the Geller children. This capacity may be directly tied with individuation and fading egocentricity.

The Eskimo value system, according to Jerome Bruner, stresses self-reliance but "strongly suppresses any expression of individualism as an attitude toward life."[3] This self-reliance depends on an unbroken relationship and rapport with the flow of nature. Thus, the Eskimo retains his primary perceptions and perceives interrelations and intricacies of his physical environment, including an airplane engine. Physical reality is reality to one who is in tune with the earth. But this is a one-way, passive reception for the Eskimo. Without some final separation of self from world, objectivity is blocked, and understanding does not follow knowing. He flows with the movement of life but cannot stand outside his action and comprehend *creating* movement out of that flow.

Once concrete operational functions have given full ability to interact with the physical processes, our intelligence should be free for formal operations, such as turning around, observing our concrete interactions, and retracing our steps to see how we did it. Then we can correlate that ability with other activity and apply it over a wide range. This is what we sometimes accomplish with our schooling, and this is what the Eskimo or Balinese fail to do perhaps because they never fully separate from the world process as individuals. Their development is arrested somewhere in a mixture of practical intelligence, as developed in the first seven years, and certain restricted forms of concrete operational intelligence.

Ordinarily, it is the opposite with us. We bring about a premature separation between self and world, lose our unity before physical survival can develop, and plunge into a fixed cultural form of formal operational thinking, the semantic reality system based on anxiety over survival. Add to this the loss, through neglect or negative feedback, of primary perceptions and bonds with the earth, and our dependency on our semantic system is doubled. In a way, we in our culture skip crucial developments from age four or five and leap ahead to restricted, concretized forms of formal operations opening around eleven or so. We say the nonliterates do not develop true individuality, but what we experience as individuality is alienation from and abandonment of the life process. Literate and nonliterate cultures represent extremes of imbalance, failures to achieve creative interaction.

In spite of our imbalances, our culture is the one holding the promise for the magical child because we can, as a result of our separation, stand back and look objectively, even at our own extreme isolation. We can retrace our steps, as Geber, Ainsworth, LeBoyer, Klaus, and a host of others are helping us do, and see what needs to be filled in so that our development might lead, not to isolation and alienation from our earth, but to creative relationships. We have the capacity to learn from the preliterate or so-called primitive culture and pick up vital qualities missing in our own without having to abandon our objectivity. In spite of institutional strangleholds on thought, we maintain avenues of open inquiry and may yet achieve a balance between nature and nurture.

Consider *suggestology,* a learning procedure developed in Bulgaria and given some rather sensational attention that detracted from its actual worth.⁴ The system has been employed in Canada and at Pepperdine College in Los Angeles but not, so far as I know, with children here. Adult students are guided in relaxation techniques and a kind of childlike play; this is accompanied by quiet, incidental music. When their inhibitions to the relaxed play have been sufficiently broken down, a subject, generally a foreign language, is quietly broadcast along with the musical background while the students concentrate only on their play. Within weeks, the students have a grasp and fluency in the language or subject.

What the procedure does is occupy the conscious, volitional self (so conditioned to be anxious and concerned over learning) in relaxed, nonpurposive play. This gets the anxious, tightly screening volitional self out of the way, freeing the vast computational abilities of the brain. The participants know a learning process is under way, but they are not called upon to work at learning, nor are they tested in any ordinary sense. They are eventually drawn into some application of their learning in a casual manner and find that the material is at their disposal.

Consider this activity from the standpoint of the learning system proposed in the earlier chapters of this book: play on the surface and work beneath that surface. In suggestology, the conscious volitional system is gotten out of the way of the work beneath by involving the person in a game activity; within weeks, a new subject is mastered without conscious work. The limitless capacity of the mind-brain for absorption and computation of new material is freed of the encumberances of a self system conditioned to believe that it must do the work of the nonconscious conceptual system.

Now consider this idea from a slightly different perspective. The maturing of intelligence should be the gradual merging and interaction between the conscious self playing on the surface and the conceptual system working beneath that surface. Colin Turnbull, in his observations of a hunting-gathering people of Africa, found that the adults play continually with the infants and children and the children play continually in the adult world. The adults make miniature utensils for the children (bows and arrows, cooking items, household gadgets such as they are) and play with the children at using them. And it is true play, the adults delighting in the child's delight at the mutual interaction. Somewhere along the line, the child moves smoothly and easily into more adult roles; the items of play grow more functional, until finally the young person is playing at reality alongside the adults. Never at any point is there a break in this progression, a point at which play becomes real. It is *all* real and *all* play.

We could do the same with a far greater range of mind and possibility if no split between work and play is arbitrarily formed. That is, if the child were allowed to play and the work allowed to unfold properly, the parallel lines of work and play would essentially merge by adulthood. In suggestology, some hint of this power is found, but something is amiss. Why should the volitional self be a hindrance to learning? Why should we have to trick our self system into getting out of the way so that the conceptual system can function? Does this not still divide the system, and is there not a strong possibility that far more profound levels of learning would be in store for us if the self system could be in synchronous flow with the conceptual system?

In spite of protestations by suggestologists that the technique has no similarity to hypnotism, there is a similarity. The student has, in effect, surrendered his volition to the experiment and the people running the venture. The student's system is divided, with ordinary consciousness not participating in the learning. This is necessary because that ordinary consciousness is locked in anxiety about learning (fear of failure, of not learning, and so on). Can we not look beyond the surface rewards of the process, though, and see a far richer reward. If the nonpersonal conceptual system can learn so fast and thoroughly, what would be the possibilities for the whole mind, if conscious volition and the inner work were in harmony? That is what nature drives for and what should unfold in late preadolescence and adolescence. Then every event in life, every unfolding moment, would be learning and, eventually, the creativity that such learning would give.

Chapter 21

Journey into the Mind:
Creative Reality

Occasionally, as I sit at my work, pouring over research papers heavy with professional jargon, I lean back, heavy-lidded, to relax for a moment. Suddenly, I am looking into a large, elaborately furnished, stately room in full dimensions. As in a slow-motion film sequence, the strange room slides past and another takes its place, then another. As easily as the imagery started, it fades and I am again pouring over a research report. Less than a minute has elapsed, yet I feel refreshed and oddly tranquil.

A friend of mine, a successful businessman, leans back in his office chair for five minutes of a total relaxation developed over the years. Suddenly, he seems to do a slow roll and finds himself apparently free of his physical body and moving, or rather floating, into unknown and rather alien territory. Involved in the ensuing events, he loses track of time, suddenly remembers an appointment, wills himself back to normal, glances at his watch, and finds that the usual five minutes have elapsed.

The great nineteenth-century scientist Kekule had long pondered certain problems of chemistry. One day, in a moment of complete relaxation, he suddenly saw clearly, right in front of him, snakes with their tales in their mouths, interlocking in a certain configuration. Kekule had the answer to his years of search. The benzene ring, the basis of modern chemistry, had been born.[1]

Albert Einstein, in his playful musings on reality (he idolized Charlie Chaplin and longed to be a great comic actor) would feel a sudden muscular twinge, an internal visceral sensation, that signaled into an illumination some vast universal principle. It then took some doing for the necessary translation of this bodily impression into linguistic form.

A young man and woman I know who attend a college in California have learned to control their night dreaming well enough to enter into each other's dreams and share them. Their independent reports, written the next morning, invariably tally.

These are only a few of the myriad types of experience available through formal operational thinking. The necessary preliminaries for such ability begin at about age eleven. At about age fifteen, the brain goes into another of its periodic cycles, with a new burst of growth and another shift of logic into full reversibility thinking and pure abstract logical ability. At the same time, with genital sexuality unfolding, the body moves toward full stature. From ages eleven to fifteen, concrete operations have been practiced and increasingly varied while abstract learning has given greater abilities for thinking about thinking. Now, at fifteen or so, with the techniques of physical survival learned and nearly autonomic, a two-pronged drive opens: genital sexuality, leading to species survival, and the journey into the mind, which leads to eventual personal survival.

Through formal operational thinking, the mind-brain can operate on its own thought processes, act back on its own functions, and change them. We are all familiar with certain concrete forms of this kind of thinking, as found in science, technology, and ordinary academic pursuits. But the creative capacity of the mind-brain ranges infinitely beyond any current use; it can synthesize its contents and create an ever larger expanse of possibility. All possible states are equally valid to this open process; any evaluations are up to us.

What we must bear in mind is that any perception we experience is the result of conceptual activity in the brain, whether that perception is of the living earth or of a benzene ring in the form of snakes. The brain can act on sensory information coming in from the world, or it can act on the sensory system and furnish perceptions originating completely within itself. Formal operational thinking can certainly act on and synthesize new ideas out of the cultural body of ideas, but it can also be a conceptual activity springing autonomously from those infinitely interacting patterns of rhythmic firing that almost never cease in the brain. Furthermore, as we found with the child's primary perceptions, those rhythmic patterns can also respond to stimuli from the primary process within the mind-brain and give equally valid perceptions. It is all reality to the experiencing mind, just as play reality and adult reality are equally real and equally arbitrary to the child.

We have been conditioned to believe that only creative thoughts arising from and contributing to our culture's arts and sciences are valid, just as we have been conditioned to believe that only perceptions arising from physical sensory stimuli are valid. Yet one of our strongest emotional-psychological needs is for the brain to give expression to its own creative capacity. We believe that a perceptual experience must be subject to consensual evaluation to be genuine, which means the source of the stimulus must be in physical reality, else it must be a hallucination and a threat to our orientation. This distrust of the brain's creativity and its ability to furnish spontaneous sensory perceptions sharply reduces the range of our intelligence and is one of the reasons we use only a portion of our brain capacity.

The mind can eventually turn to its own brain's processes, stand outside those computations, and operate on them to change them and so change the resulting information. That continual refinement can eventually separate thinker from thinking so that the thinker can create ideas out of ideas and create imaginative patterns for concrete operations that earlier had to have models for suggestion. Then the mind-brain can represent some aspect of reality metaphorically and amass critical groups of related ideas.

This action between volitional choice and primary process is how we arrive at any kind of answer, intellectual, scientific, creative, or spiritual. The great thrust of modern man has been to question how he received his answers; we desire to know how our solutions are achieved, and this involves full reversibility thinking in its academic sense: the ability not only to achieve a solution but also to retrace our steps in creating that solution.

All creativity is an expression of reversibility thinking. Historically, we have assumed that the only continuum of possibility is one generated by the physical world around us, for otherwise how can possibilities be developed and shared with others? But this has led to human creativity being limited to *mediated* forms; that is, creativity has been expressed only through some material means of transference from one mind-brain to another. Immediately, in fact, we wonder how there can be any other kind of creativity. The word itself causes trouble. When we think of a creative child, we tend to think of crayon and paper, daubs of clay, perhaps a flute, and an overall indulgence. When we think of an intellectual child, we think of mathematics, books, chemistry sets, and practical, real things. Both are obviously areas of creativity, expressions of the ability to interact with possibilities.

In fantasy play, the child sees a truck or boat in the matchbox, and chooses his/her possibility from a continuum in the same way Michelangelo saw the finished statute in the rough stone. The child transforms the real matchbox into his/her play-reality boat and enters into that reality. Michelangelo transformed the stone itself into his imagined picture of it. The child's transformed reality has no consensus value; s/he experiences his/her creation alone. Michelangelo's transformation is available on a consensual level, and we enjoy it for centuries. What the child transforms is unchanged; the return is to the unchanged point of origin. The stone is never again the same once Michelangelo uses the medium of tools to express his creativity through the medium of the stone. The statue is an aspect of the earth plus the human mind expressing itself through a physical tool. Thus, it is a form of abstraction out of concreteness, or concrete operational thinking; whereas the child's fantasy reality is an aspect of the earth plus mind without any intermediary devices.

Science and its technology and all art must be expressed through concrete mediums. Even mathematics and music, which are closest to pure abstractions, must be expressed through the medium of symbols or signs if they are to be communicated. There are mathematical geniuses who can do great computations in their heads, but they must revert to some kind of medium to express themselves to others. Mozart conceived his works in gestalt form, experiencing them as complete units. His labor came in translating that inner perfection into the digital, linear signs other musicians could interpret and so give the music life.

An art form is a medium of expression, and the medium determines the art. The wonder of the human mind is that such mediums of translation can be invented and that such wide uses of these inventions then evolve. The great difference between Western and Eastern music rests on the West's invention of musical notation. The medium of idea transference created wide new dimensions for musical creativity itself, just as mathematical symbols added vast dimensions beyond counting on toes and fingers, the printing press created the Gutenberg galaxy, the medium becomes the message, and so on.

Consider, though, that the maturation of intelligence is programmed to move from concreteness toward greater abstraction or pure thought. No matter how pure, formal, and abstract our formal operational thought becomes, even in our purest scientific research, we must express it through some form of concreteness, some medium of translation and transference. That is, all art and science is an expression of mature thought that must nevertheless use intermediary materials. We might say that the stage of development opening at adolescence seems always to have to be expressed through the stage opening at age seven.

All our creativity, then, has so far been a combination of formal and concrete thinking, and this is surely one of the great combinational forms available to us. But with due respect, awe, and wonder for this kind of creation, I would point out that it is limited, nevertheless, to the concreteness of its medium. The mature intelligence should be able to interact with the possibilities of the living earth, that living earth plus the creativity of the mind, and the processes and products of the mind-brain itself. So far, we have used this third category of possibility only in relation to the second category. That is, the mind-brain has not become its own matrix, as planned genetically for the period of late adolescence and maturity.

Any artist will tell you that the medium of the art is the hurdle that must be overcome in order for creativity to unfold. The pianist performing 800 individual strokes per minute must get beyond the notes to get to the music. Surely the same applies to all art forms and even the sciences. The issue is that great creative thought can arise only from the proper concrete background; the progression is never violated.

What, then, would be a truly mature form of creativity? It would be one of pure abstractions that did not require concrete forms of expression. Although this pure development could take place only through the disciplined learning of tangible, material forms, such unmediated creativity would be the highest thrust of human intelligence. The medium of transfer for this formal, abstract act of creation would be (and is) the primary process. Being the common factor of every mind-brain, the primary process can be the medium for expression of pure creation. The creative formation itself is also of the primary process, and the creative receptors are the individual expressions of that process: you and me. One of us can create a pure abstraction in his or her head and through the primary process which participates in that creation can share the resulting perceptions with someone else. And that is one aspect of the mind-brain becoming its own matrix.

Unmediated creativity is quite common. Ordinary dreams are a form of unmediated creation. Unstable and crude as the perceptions generally are, we are still perceiving in dreams, and this means conceptual activity in the brain. The undisciplined and chaotic nature of such experience is probably the fault, not of the function, but of its lack of education and organizing. In lucid dreams, we get closer to a reversible type of controlled perceptions, we suddenly recognize that we are dreaming and find that we can maintain some control and a kind of ordinary consciousness in them. We are at that point standing outside brain computations and directing their flow.

The brain churns in continuous activity with apparently more noise than signals; that is, much brain action is unproductive. This is particularly true of daydreaming and roof-brain chatter. In fact, we spend most of our waking state in this unreal energy attention and attend the mechanics of existence only peripherally. Thus, the magical thinking of the child carries right over into adult life. But whereas the child believes his/her magical thinking to be the truth and anticipates coming into his/her powers to implement it, we adults recognize our daydream and internal chatter to be only safety valves of fulfillment that make reality more bearable.

We are geared, not for tedium, but for novelty. The infant grows through novelty and likes complex patterns better than plain ones. We quickly screen out the humdrum and look for something different. Repetitiveness is dullness. Generally, our escape is through daydreaming and internal conversations. The creativity of the mind-brain has many other possibilities as well, but although we look for novelty, we look for it in restricted, safe, and rather nonnovel ways.

The hypnagogic state is an example of our creative possibilities, but we are the recipients of this creative action. My only control or part in the state is to remain absolutely passive and receptive. This experience takes place at some halfway point between sleep and wakefulness. It bears some resemblance to lucid dreaming in its utter visual and often aural clarity and spatial characteristics.[2] At moments of awakening from a brief nap while working or early in the morning when I am sitting quietly, my mind pauses at some house halfway to common reality, and I receive quite lovely gifts. I call them gifts because I have nothing to do about them other than receiving them. When consciousness returns, but the sensory system remains shut down for a brief moment or so, other kinds of perceptions pour in, as my creativity leaps into the temporary void, delighted with the chance to play with me. One morning, for instance, I was up at 2:00 A.M. A field mouse had decided to take up quarters with me and began busily gnawing new runway entrances and exits. (I don't know why; there must have been several hundred perfectly good ones all over the cabin.) He made such an infernal din, in spite of my pounding, pleading, and threatening, that I finally gave up, dressed, lit the lamp, and started working on this chapter. About dawn, I grew drowsy and blew out the lamp. As I watched the light grow stronger, my eyes rested on my large brick fireplace, and as it turned out, I suppose, I then closed my eyes. Immediately, without transition, I was still looking at bricks, still in apparent three dimensions, but I became aware of an enormous sweep of brick wall—not a building's wall, but a huge interior wall, with niches and ornamentations. The whole sweep had an exciting threshold-of-discovery feeling, and I realized that I had swung into a hypnagogic state triggered by the bricks of my fireplace. At that point of self-conscious awareness, the scene faded (to my disappointment, since some enormous discovery had seemed imminent), and I found myself staring at my own fireplace. The usual posthypnagogic feelings of peace, security, warmth, luxuriousness, power, and confidence flooded me, and I forgot my disappointment over the brevity of the incident.

For a period of a year or more, most of my hypnagogic experiences centered on rooms. At night on going to bed, or early on first awakening, or catnapping, I would suddenly find myself observing rooms, again without apparent transition from ordinary wakefulness. Whole series of extraordinary rooms would simply file by in three dimensions, rooms of every conceivable form. Sometimes, they flowed in stately procession; at other times, faster and faster, until I no more than glimpsed each as a whizzing blur. Sometimes, the sequences of rooms unfolded vertically, from bottom up; but most of the time, they moved from left to right. Generally, I could view the rooms only as though from one side; but on a few memorable occasions, I managed to stop the flow and enter them. At that point, the experience seemed to blend into lucid dreaming. Once, and only once, I met occupants of a room that way and had a truly hilarious time with them. They were not exactly human characters, but quite dreamlike. They agreed with me that I was dreaming them but said it made no difference because they were also dreaming me, which struck us all as funny beyond words, and we roared with laughter. Then, I could hold the room no longer and felt myself melting through the floor (the sequence had been unfolding vertically). We shouted our good-byes, and they made me promise to come back. Alas, such control is not mine. I came out of the state still laughing.

The esoteric and occult schools would claim I had been traveling around, but I doubt this is the case. I was simply being given perceptions to enjoy by my creative primary process, which had an infinite amount of this sort of play rather going to waste. A year or so ago, I had the most impressive of hypnagogic experiences. Early one morning, I awoke and arose immediately (I do not enjoy lying in bed after I awake). Others of my family were up, and I heard kitchen rattling and banging. Immediately, though, I had an overpowering urge to lie down and close my eyes, which I did, recognizing the onset of a hypnagogic experience. My senses remained at least partially alert throughout this venture, which was quite unusual; and at one point, someone came in, saying that they had thought I was up. I replied with such an explosive *"SHH"* that they immediately desisted and the state went unbroken, which was even more unusual because the hypnagogic state is as fragile as a soap bubble.

Immediately after closing my eyes, I thought a brilliant light must have been turned on my closed lids, for I saw a great red field, as though of brilliant red velvet, that was three-dimensional and had a vast depth extending to cover the whole universal field. This red velvet universe was exquisitely beautiful for some reason, with heavy numinous overtones; that is, it was tinged with religious awe and wonder. Just as I was coming to grips with the astonishing dimensions and qualities of this experience, fragile horizontal gold lines appeared in neat symmetrical parallels in the immediate foreground. The effect of the brilliant gold lines against the red was stunning, and I all but wept at the sight. Then, in neat and slow procession, vertical gold lines appeared behind the horizontal in perfect parallel precision, and behind these another set of horizontals, and so on, until the universal field seemed a magnificent grid of gold against red, giving the panorama great sweep and depth. By then, I had the feeling of being in deep space that hypnagogic imagery often gives. Finally, as though simply to demonstrate in casual beauty the powers of creation being tendered me, appeared a luminous green sphere of light on each gold line, the gold line directly through its center. Each globe, an unearthly iridescent green, then began a slow and stately movement along its respective gold line stretching away through the universe of red.

When it faded, I shouted aloud, "No! No!" Of course, I wanted to stay there forever. It was nice, better than TV. For weeks afterward, the effect lingered within me, the warm luxury of unity and power mixed with a strange longing or homesickness. I had been given a gift, and I like to think it has not been wasted.

One might wonder if this is not illusion, hallucination, or delirium. Have I seen my analyst lately? Ah, I reply, if this be madness, let me never regain sanity. And what is such an experience good for? True, the experience seems worthless. I cannot package it and sell it, nor even duplicate it. Nor, in case the reader wonders, is it related to drugs; I do not take them. I am given gifts (as we all are) by that great work beneath my surface. All I am asked to do is to receive, to play.

Nor are our gifts limited to experiences of a sensory nature of this sort. Many of them, coming at night in high, cosmic dreams, in prayer, in meditation, or simply off moments of blankness, have no basis in ordinary sensory awareness and so cannot be described. These gifts are ineffable, as they say, and, although the most powerful of all, not even available to recall of content.

Creations of the mind-brain that could be shared by people is my concern for now. Note that the hypnagogic experiences I have related were perceived by me as clearly as my ordinary daily world, if not far more clearly. When I glanced at those geometric drawings and my body-parked friends immediately perceived them, our perceptions were shared through our primary process, that hologram of unified experience. The shared item was a material object, graphite on paper, and yet had nowhere near the depth, clarity, significance, and power of my hypnagogic experience. Theoretically, it must then be biologically and psychologically feasible to share a hypnagogic kind of creativity with another mind. Indeed, there are an array of legitimate experiments along just such a line.

Recall Charles Tart's two subjects in the telepathic experiment, when B was shocked and A's body-knowing clearly stated when the shocks occurred even though A as a conscious person was not aware of the event. Very clearly, A's mind-brain picked up from B's experience without any medium of exchange other than the mechanisms of mind-brain, which includes the medium of the primary process, mediating an actual occurrence between two people.

The same effect can be brought about when the only point of departure is pure imagination or creativity originating in one mind-brain and picked up and shared by another. And when two mind-brain systems share the same created experience, that experience becomes consensual between those two, a common property of the senses of both, in the same way a semantic cultural reality does among millions of people, and agreement on a common property of shared senses immediately stabilizes the sensory information.

For example, Dr. Tart developed a system for mutual hypnosis.[3] Two of his graduate assistants, a young man and a young woman, were very good at giving large-scale tests for hypnotic susceptibility. And they proved to be very good hypnotic subjects themselves. Tart trained the young woman to put the young man under hypnosis and then command the young man to put *her* under. Tart kept himself in rapport with both to give each the suggestion to further the other's hypnotic depth and to keep himself as the objective observer ready to intercede if unforeseen problems arose.

To be put under hypnosis, that young man had to surrender his volitional choice system and, in effect, give it over to the young woman. At that point, she became his capacity to choose what his primary process should furnish as his created reality. The young woman then had to suspend her volitional choice system and give it over to the young man to be hypnotized herself. So each had surrendered the choice system to the other, and the choice factors of their brain computers at that point became a kind of mutually shared system.

The result was that the techniques they were using to induce deeper hypnosis in the other, back and forth, at some critical point became conceptual reality for them. For instance, the boy was instructing the girl to imagine a tunnel into which they were going down deeper into hypnosis. At that point, he had chosen some specific concrete reality patterning for her conceptual system to organize around, and it complied with quite realistic sensory perceptions of a tunnel for her. She then used the same imagery, now quite vivid for her, to induce further depth to his hypnotic state. And, as in our group experiments when I had looked at geometric drawings and these had transferred to the group, suddenly the boy and girl were together in the tunnel. At the moment the tunnel imagery was mutually shared and given consensus between them, that tunnel took on full-dimensional sensory reality. It smelled, felt, looked, and sounded like a regular tunnel. They could distinguish no difference in the reality of the tunnel and the reality of any ordinary daily event in the actual world. They knew, of course, that the affair was not real, yet they finally terminated the experience because the tunnel's realness was as great as any other and they became anxious to reestablish the real reality of their everyday world. They had chosen and granted validity to a state from a continuum of possible states, entertained that state as reality, but then felt the need to return to the point from which the operation of mind began.

Since the details of the tunnel were shared and identical, they began conversing with each other in that created state, rather than using their actual voices there in their ordinary reality, where Tart was trying to remain in rapport with them. He continually got left out. Another graduate assistant came in, however, sat down, and being an excellent subject, quickly fell into hypnosis. She found herself in the pair's tunnel; they sensed her presence and resented it; the tunnel, was, after all, their thing. She sensed their resentment and retreated to a far part of the tunnel, where she watched unobserved.

On another occasion, the pair used the metaphor of a golden rope up which they were climbing to reach deeper states of hypnosis. The girl found the rope hard to climb and switched to a golden rope ladder. Suddenly, the pair found themselves on a magnificent golden beach, with a champagne ocean, crystal rocks, heavenly choirs singing overhead. The experience was so unexpected, awesome, and majestic that they held hands to give each other courage. Every item of their created state had stabilized because it was shared. They could taste, touch, smell, and hear as they could in everyday life. The phenomena did not shift, as such things do in a dream. On one occasion, they turned toward each other unexpectedly, occupied the same physical space, at which point their personal identities merged, each perceived him/herself as their combined personalities. This was unnerving. The boy insisted they leave the state and count down to normal.

The young man was so unnverved by the series of experiments that he refused to continue. He could no longer grant himself consensus about what was really real because the nonordinary reality that they had mutually created and shared was sensorally the same as his everyday experience.

An unexpected result (to which we will return in Chapter 22) was that the boy and girl very quickly developed a puzzling deep affinity for each other. They could not bear being separated during the weeks of the experiments. Jean Houston, whose Foundation for Mind Research delves into phenomena of this sort, warns against using mixed couples or pairs in mutual hypnosis unless those pairs are prepared for deep emotional involvement.

A group of friends and I found that in deep hypnotic states, one member of the group could begin a hypnotic dream, when so directed by the guide, and others would quickly find themselves both experiencing and contributing to that dream. The minute two or more were sharing the dream, it stabilized and became an ordinary consensus reality available to all the senses. These states then seemed permanent; the group could return to them later, as could the individual members of the group.

A college student related having lost three years to LSD addiction. He and a friend had tripped together regularly, until they finally shared all their states. On one occasion, they asked another friend to stay around and watch after them while they tripped. The friend was a poetic, religious, and intellectual person who would not experiment with drugs or alcohol. In proximity to them, however, he got caught up in their created state and tripped right along with them. They were surprised to find their baby-sitter in their LSD state, and he was equally surprised—and delighted. All three partook of the adventure and, on returning to normal, wrote out their accounts; the accounts were the same.

Robert Monroe is a successful businessman who made a fortune through television and radio stations. Through a number of chance events, he experienced leaving his physical body a number of years ago. This happens to many people once and briefly, but Monroe was adventurous, astute, and brave enough to develop the experience until it became commonplace for him. *Exteriorization* is the ordinary term for a person having the perception of leaving his body and being a free mind agent (although it may be a misnomer, as is "out of the body"). The esoteric disciplines call it *astral travel.* Some of Tart's early work at the University of Virginia Medical Hospital involved making electroencephalic tracings of epileptic and severe migraine patients. He found that they often apparently separated from their bodies when in the depths of a seizure. A young professor from Leeds

University in England came to the University of North Carolina at Chapel Hill a number of years ago, and found that his graduate students could, under deep hypnosis, be commanded to leave their bodies, in effect, and give reports on other professors in other offices about the campus, or even on events far away. The students could give quite accurate reports, easily verifiable by telephone. The famous psychic Edgar Cayce could do something similar while in deep trance. He called it temporarily inhabiting someone's body. If given a target person's name and address, he could give reportedly accurate accounts of that person's activities. In the 1840s, a Maine shoemaker, Phineas Quimby, could locate missing people this way and reportedly healed people by inhabiting their bodies, assuming their illness for them, and returning to his own healthy body to throw off the illness. (Many shaman follow this procedure for healing.)

Drs. Targ and Puthoff, of Stanford Research Institute, both reputable laser scientists with many patents behind them, have recently produced an interesting effect of a similar nature. Subjects, including hitherto non-psychic Stanford professors, sit in a Faraday cage (which screens out radio waves or other means for fraud) and give (often to their great surprise) accurate reports of unknown target areas being visited by one of the researchers at that moment. The researcher is given a sealed envelope containing the name of the target area to be visited and goes to look around that target area while the subject in the Faraday cage relaxes and reports any impressions that arise in his mind. In a majority of cases, these impressions are of the target area. Targ and Puthoff have run some fifty-five people, including scientists and other professionals, through the system with astonishing results.

However, Robert Monroe's experiences are probably the most intriguing of any person's in our time, with the possible exception of Carlos Castaneda's. And Robert Monroe proves to have the same astonishing courage we find in Castaneda's accounts. I urge everyone to read Monroe's *Journeys Out of the Body*, in which he gives a calm, analytic, and nonsensational account of his bizarre and at times terrible experiences. I will give only two examples here, neither being typical of the esoteric events he eventually found himself in (and still does). On one occasion, while Monroe was apparently out of his body, he visited old friends, came back, and gave an accurate account of their condition, including the friend's new illness (unknown until that moment) and other details. He had, of course, not left his office. On another occasion, he "visited" friends and was determined to make them notice him (no one ever saw him when he exteriorated, but he saw them). When no one paid him the slightest attention (and he had traveled hundreds of miles in seconds to pay them a call), he pinched the lady involved very hard on her bottom. The lady did not see him, but she felt the pinch so keenly that she screamed aloud; and the pinch left an all-too-real large blue bruise, as a telephone conversation later that day revealed.

What makes Monroe's experience so credible is the man himself: an eminently sane, sensible, and warm person, extremely successful in the business world. Above all, he has developed, in his electronics laboratories, an astonishing system for helping people to duplicate his own feats; it works. Elizabeth Kubler-Ross, a Swiss psychiatrist and author, underwent his training and had such an overwhelming experience that she now works in this field.

When we have the impression of leaving our bodies, we are probably really entering the total hologram of the primary process. Our conceptual system can process stimuli from this field only as it finds points of similarity, but occasionally, one stumbles into stimuli that have no such points, and massive confusion and disorientation occur. Rather than "out of the body," these ventures should be more aptly called "into the mind." Most of us, exteriorizing in this fashion accidentally (which happens at least once to most people), are terrorized beyond all measure and throw up such barriers to a repeat performance that it never happens again. I am sure that these chance happenings are attempts at establishing our bonds to a final matrix shift.

One night, I underwent a severe tachycardia attack. (The ventricals of the heart go out of rhythmic phase, so that the left ventrical pumps before the other opens, and they get quite chaotic.) In such an attack, blood loss to the brain brings on faintness, and the heart starts working harder. Big thumpings seem to jump against your esophagus, and you feel that you are passing out. The affair is no fun. Overcoming the panic (I had earlier had a similar attack), I began a slow, rhythmic deep breathing and concentration to keep my heart rate stable and slowed down, a technique I had picked up in yoga meditation.

It was past midnight, and I kept falling to sleep, my body jerking me awake in panic as my heart derailed again. So I gingerly got up, went down to the living room, where sleep connotations were not so rife, turned on the lights, and sat bolt upright on the sofa to continue the stabilizing routine. Suddenly, I seemed to be doing a slow somersault right out into the middle of the room. There I was, free as a bird, floating about. Ecstatic, I went swooping about in typical flying-dream style while my poor physical part sat there on the sofa, eyes staring straight ahead, doing rhythmic breathing.

I thought of taking off somewhere, and it was no sooner said than done. At that point (according to my later analysis, at least), the venture phased into a high-lucid dream because it took on the characteristics of both hypnagogic and lucid-dream states. I was flying down a beautiful path in a lovely garden (bright daylight, of course, not 1:00 A.M. and pitch-black), only to be beset with unbearable, anguished sexual desire (a common phenomenon according to Robert Monroe, whom I had not then heard of). The beautiful state instantly complied with this, too, and there in that lavish place appeared surely the most beautiful and enticing female that ever graced one's senses. She was smiling, beckoning. Just when I should have responded to that lovely creature, I suddenly remembered that I was really sitting there in the living room, trying to keep my heart stable. I underwent a moment of extremely anguished indecision, convinced that if I responded to that lovely person, with this wretched self here, I would surely never return to that mundane living room. That tachycardia would have the last word. My concern for my motherless offspring flooded me and won out, and instantly there I was, sitting on the couch, staring into the room, counting (inhale for eight, hold for four, exhale for eight; again).

Wilder Penfield made the observation, after some fifty years of brain research, that mind and brain share the same organizational processes but are not synonymous phenomena. Mind receives its energy from brain and, in turn, acts as kind of director general over the intent and operations of that brain. Penfield claims that mind has no memory. It does not need memory because it has its computer; it can simply push the memory button and get what is needed.

What then is mind? As we have seen, it is intent preceding ability in the infant, simply impulse toward content. But content is incidental to this intent, except as a way of development, a way of learning to interact. So I propose that mind is the ability to interact itself, with what is incidental. Intelligence is the muscular-mindedness to enter into and experience an ever wider field of possibility, which is at the same time the ability to create that possibility out of the continuum of possibility.

In the admittedly esoteric examples offered in this chapter, I have given the materials by which creativity in one's own mind-brain might be shared directly with another mind-brain and, in that sharing, organize a mutually held reality experience. Such shared reality offers full sensory stimuli, feedback, stability, and open-endedness, which means other possibilities can then spill off that state if one has the muscular-mindedness to hold and go farther. The shared state then offers a new source of energy, possibility, and safe space; the matrix has then become fluid and open, as life planned. This is autonomy of the person.

The brain, however, is a material organization. It is of the same concrete stuff as matrix earth. The movement of intelligence is from this concreteness toward abstraction. Penfield observed that the brain, after age forty or so, starts losing something like 100,000 cells a day. This may not be an immediate problem; the brain probably acts as a hologram, in that cells themselves begin to reflect the structure of the whole system. (We know you can remove large chunks of the adult brain without much impairment.) Nevertheless, Penfield noted that as he grew older, his computer did not work so well. Memory was not so readily there at the push of the button; computations slowed down. Speaking from his eightieth year, however, Penfield also noted that the slower the old computer got, the brighter and quicker the mind grew.

Mind is the ability to interact. The content through which this ability develops is, as you see, inconsequential. The fall of the developing child is in his/her being conditioned to believe that it is the content of interaction that is important. S/he begins to seize content as a buffer to anxiety, a kind of lifelong search for one security blanket after another. The magical child is one whose ability is his/her focus and who does not lose him/herself to content or memory.

Considering the brain as a hologram, we have an answer to Alfred North Whitehead's puzzling statement: "There is a way in which all things are in all places at the same time." He has described the way the brain acts as a hologram of an earth which is a hologram of larger holograms. This functions in us as a primary process, which, as the sum of all things, may well incorporate our personal history, giving us our uniqueness. In his closing statements, Penfield theorized that if mind could ever be found to receive its energy from any source other than its own brain, we would then know that personal survival is possible after the brain's destruction. I have given selected examples from a wide range of possibilities that show conclusively that one mind-brain can be powered by another mind-brain and that the mind-brain can be powered by the primary process itself.

Judging from the whole thrust of development, in its movement from concreteness toward abstraction, logic impels us to consider that the final step of autonomy is for mind to become its own matrix. Nothing exists except as an interchange of energy. The primary process, mind at large, must then be the matrix with which mind, separated from brain, relates. Nature never provides for a matrix shift without providing ample bondings with that new matrix ahead of time. Such bondings between mind and mind are the concerns of a much later stage, beyond the scope of a book on the child. They are the concerns of a vast literature from yogic and Sufic traditions and, more recently and indirectly, from Elizabeth Kubler-Ross.

Chapter 22

The Second Bonding:
Yin and Yang

In the 1940s, biologists discovered what one woman called the best-kept male chauvinist secret in the history of biology, centering on the fact that the male sperm can be of either an X- or a Y-chromosome construction, whereas the female egg is always an X chromosome. The Y-chromosome sperm is much faster and stronger than the X sperm and nearly always wins the race to the egg. But the Y sperm is also quite short-lived, and unless the egg is right there, ready and waiting, the swift sperm quickly dies. The weaker and slower X sperm arrives later and, being of a more stable nature, can hang around a bit if the egg is not ready. If the X sperm succeeds in penetrating the X egg, an X-chromosome embryo will develop, which means a female embryo. If the Y-chromosome sperm wins out, an XY-chromosome embryo results, which means a male embryo—maybe. The success of this XY embryo depends upon the balanced production of the hormone testosterone. If this hormone production is not successful, the embryo's XY-chromosome structure reverts back to an X status somewhere between the sixth and eighth embryonic week. That which would have been male returns to a female structure, or it aborts or grows into a confused gender, not quite male or female.

This discovery indicated that the base line of organic life is essentially female, with the production of a male subject to some inherent risk. Ashley

Montagu's studies showed that about 50 percent of all human fertilizations seem to abort spontaneously somewhere between the sixth and eighth embryonic weeks. Most such women, Montagu surmised, are unaware that they have, in fact, conceived. They simply miss a period or even two, and suddenly all is normal again.

Another stage of spontaneous natural abortion occurs around the fifth month, probably because the massive undifferentiated brain-cell growth begins its differentiation into functioning organs during this period. At any rate, a majority of these fifth-month abortions will be male fetuses. A certain number of infants are born prematurely around the seventh month, and a majority of these will be males. Of normal nine-month deliveries, a percentage will be defective (blind, deaf, malformed in some way). Some 80 percent of these will be males; 80 percent of all silent crib deaths are males; and 80 percent of all autistic children are males (and 80 percent of these will be firstborn males); 80 percent of schizophrenic, hyperactive, retarded, and generally dysfunctional children will be males. Male births outnumber female births, yet mature females outnumber males.

Consider, then, that if the production of testosterone is incomplete, the XY embryo will revert to an X embryo to some degree or abort. If Montagu's observations are correct, then, by simple logic, we can see that probably 80 percent of these abortions will be unsuccessful males. Apparently, nature has to try far more frequently to produce a male, and he is much more subject to natural selection. Beneath his postures, stances, and gestures of defiance, the male somehow perhaps senses this and is more prone to anxiety than the female.

Infant monkeys were separated from their mothers in childhood. The male children went through some twelve hours of frenetic searching for the mother, continually giving the distress cry of separation. After this intense stress, the male monkey child collapsed into a fetal position and went into an anaclitic depression from which he would not have survived without intervention. These male children began, after some seven or eight days, to make a slow return to some normality. Their return was only partial at best, however; they proved incapable of social interaction and were sexually impotent, withdrawn, and self-destructive.

Little girl monkeys, when separated from their mothers, underwent the same intensive twelve-hour search. At the end of that time, not having found their mothers, they made an immediate return to apparent normality, with no anaclitic depression and collapse. (They later proved to be quite poor mothers and mistreated their offspring.)

Studies of human children indicate the same response. Little boys whose mothers die or abandon them suffer more emotional havoc and permanent scars than little girls do. This was the case with my own family. My two girls were four and twelve when their mother died, and they showed far fewer emotional scars than my boys, seven and nine. The studies of Massie, Zaslow and Breger, and others, strongly suggest that failure of bonding with the mother or a conditional, insufficient bonding is a frequent cause of infantile autism, but this is the case with four times as many boys as with girls. Gardner, in his study of early dwarfism, found male children the most common victims, the reason generally being the mother's unexpressed hostility toward the father unconsciously reflecting in failure to nurture the male infant physically.

Movies were shown to eight- and nine-year-old boys and girls. At moments of tension, when terrible things were about to happen on the screen, the little boys jumped up in agitation and thrust their arms out as if to fend off the disaster. The little girls sank quietly back into their chairs, grew very still, and waited. From the beginning, the female, being of the base-line genetic structuring of life, is able to flow with, bide her time, and survive. From the beginning, the male is anxious, tries to fight against, dominate, pit himself against the odds. He seems born already functionally separated from the life force that somehow underlies the female in unbroken flow. As such, he cannot survive, at least not at all well, without the female.

The unmarried adult male does very poorly compared with his married brethren (regardless of how the married brother gripes). The unmarried male has far more accidents, murders other males and is murdered by them more frequently, commits suicide far more frequently, and is ill much more often than his married brethren. And, of course, males outnumber females in such destructive actions by 10 to 1. Finally, the unmarried male has a much shorter life span than the married male; whereas the unmarried female gets along surprisingly well. She lives just as long as her married counterpart.

Psychology Today published a study showing that male intelligence was quite superior to female intelligence. Males, the study said, produce far more great geniuses, scientists, heads of states and corporations, inventors, composers, creative minds. If we accept intelligence as the ability to interact with the culture's body of knowledge, institutions, and capacity for tool production and rape of the living earth, that report would be valid. But if we accept intelligence as the ability to interact, without qualification, then the report is seriously mistaken. Certainly, a bell curve graph of intelligence shows more males at the extremely brilliant end, but it also shows far more males at the complete-catastrophe end. The excellence seems bought at a high price. Female intelligence, according to this male standard, appears as a kind of flat-line projection, neither bright nor dull, just stable.

All of this is nonsense. We have no notion of what intelligence is or what it is designed to do. Above all, we do not know what the mysterious difference between male and female intelligence is all about. What is in the quality of female intelligence, as the ability to interact, that is so vital that selection keeps this base line intact? What stability is there that makes this organism able to survive so much better that life must produce far fewer of her kind to achieve an approximate balance with the male? And what is the quality in this X base-line organism that is so terribly vital to the male? It is not just sexual attraction, for if it was, our massive preoccupation with sex would immediately solve the problem. What is the quality of male intelligence that makes nature spend so much extra effort in production trying to make the difficult balancing feat work out right? What specialty of intelligence did nature have in mind here? And, again, what is the factor missing in the male that makes him so dependent on the female?

At issue is the unbonded male child or the insufficiently bonded male. His need of bonding is biologically crucial, and the biological structure resulting from insufficient bonding is a warped, nonnatural biological organism. This thrust of nature simply goes haywire when unbonded, rather like a wild electron that has no orbit to give its energy organization, meaning, and purpose. There is something in the female that he must have from the beginning. Missing this, his machinery gets thrown out of balance. The unbonded female might become neurotic and be unable to bond to her child properly, but the unbonded male goes very subtly mad. Unless rooted to that mother matrix, his other matrices cannot form, and his machinery loses its balancing mechanism, its governor. He runs amok. What the unbonded male does is spend his life turning back on that matrix, trying to force from it that which is lacking. And what is lacking is his source of personal power, his possibility, and his safe space. Lacking these, he turns and uses his strength to rape. He rapes either crudely or with sophistication, that is, bodily, or intellectually, raping the earth matrix with technology. And he then has the chutzpah to set up an entire cultural criteria system for judging intelligence according to how successful one is in this rape of matrix. It is no surprise that in this criteria scheme, the female, who is not driven to self-rape, shows up quite poorly.

The difference between the drive for the rape of the physical body of a particular woman and of the physical body of the living earth is only a difference of degree (perhaps a college degree). The same imbalance is at root. The nonbonded male has no safe space and turns to force this from the matrix. To dominate her becomes his passion, to violate her if need be to win from her that elusive magical nutrient every female seems to have but which the unbonded male cannot get or beat out of her. Jean MacKellar makes it clear that sexual hunger has little to do with why men rape. Nor does sexual attractiveness in its usual social sense play a role; the eighty-year-old woman is just as liable to be raped as the twenty-year-old. The rapist himself does not understand the real hunger that drives him.

Our current graphs of intelligence indicate grave imbalances, not what nature intends. A true graph of male-female intelligence would not show a bell curve of wild extremes for the male and a dull, flat line for the female. In this kind of split, everyone loses. The true graph of male-female intelligence would, instead, come out looking like the double helix, a pair bond identical yet different, coiled together yet separate, neither able to function well without the other, both functioning through the bonds linking their life coils for energy interaction.

Consider the overall development of intelligence during the three stages of growth that I have outlined. The same cycle of competence that underlies any single act of learning also underlies this overall development. The first seven years rough in a knowledge of the living earth matrix to which we should bond at our individuation around age seven; the second seven years fill in the details of this knowledge of being, the details being the interactions between self and earth matrix; the final part of the cycle, probably only beginning in the next seven years, from adolescence to maturity, is the stage of practice and variation, practicing the interactions with the possibilities roughed in and filled in during the first fourteen or fifteen years. What is the ideal way to perfect and practice one's learning? To teach what one has learned. And nature provides that the magical child, as s/he approaches maturity, should perfect his/her learning by becoming a parent, which is to become the teacher of the next magical child.

The first bonding was to the earth. The second bonding is through the double helix male-female pair bond. In the wonderful economy of nature, many functions are fulfilled in this second bonding. We are a threefold organism, consisting of body, mind-brain, and something variously referred to as spirit or soul and which I have represented here as the primary process. We find this expressed in the triune nature of the brain itself: a purely physical brain system of body-knowing, an intermediary kind of brain I have called primary process, and the high brain of the self system or individuality. The progression is from the concreteness of the purely physical kind of knowing toward the purely mental, and the primary process is always the functional matrix out of which the progression springs and on which it rests.

Between the ages of eleven and fifteen, the magical child's matrix shifts to the self, a mind-brain in a body. S/he becomes his/her own source of power, possibility, and safe place, though always resting on the larger earth matrix. But the progression of concreteness toward abstraction demands that mind-brain become the new matrix by maturity. This entails a functional, logical shift of pure thinking away from body-knowing, and the logic of differentiation provides this through feedback. But no organism can exist except through interchange of energy because existence depends on flow. So for mind-brain to become its own matrix, where pure thought can detach from physical considerations, that mind-brain must relate to another mind-brain. And this, also, is what the second bonding provides. The male mind-brain bonds to and interacts with the female mind-brain for the expression of the mind-brain's vast creativity (as I outlined in Chapter 21). At the same time, this bonding allows a meshing of the primary process of the male and the female, through which nonphysical reality creations and stabilizations are possible. This gives the initial step toward mind eventually bonding with the primary process for personal survival. And finally, in the second bonding, genital sexuality gives the bonding of the physical bodies and eventually species survival in producing the next generation of the magical child. In becoming the teachers of the new magical child (which can only be done through physical-mental modeling), the parents then practice, perfect, and learn to vary their own developmental knowledge of being. It is a neat system.

When the parenting stage is over, preparations for the final matrix shift should get under way, the shift toward mind becoming its own matrix. This means that mind must functionally separate from the concrete operations of the brain. Mind can do this only by relating with another mind for the necessary energy flow, and male-female bonding should provide this. The medium would again be the primary process, mind at large. Finally, mind, or personality, can relate solely with the primary process and so be able to function independently of the physical body, brain, or world. Thus, when the life cycle as we know it ends, the next matrix shift, to mind at large, will have been properly prepared, the bonds secured. Our 3-billion-year thrust toward this has left nothing out. The matrix is always there. We always have somewhere to go if the proper bonding has taken place. The second bonding incorporates all these transitions, and so is one of the most awesome and profound experiences of life, stage-specific to late adolescence and early maturity. Generally, this great movement is thwarted by anxiety and ends in dust and ashes, but its deep and universal significance is sensed by all of us at one time or another. Just as many of us spend our lives searching for that missing matrix of mother earth, so we spend our lives looking for that love the second bonding is meant to hold. As usual, we are stalemated in the physical and concrete, searching in it for that great missing mind-spirit element. Somewhere in our broken hearts, we have always sensed this, though we have so poor an understanding of where and how it all went wrong.

Chapter 23

Renewing the Promise

At the end of a magical child seminar, I have frequently been asked: "Okay, what do we adults do now about our child and our own split selves?" All of us like prescriptions, some step-by-step spelling out of actions we should follow. Although attractive, this is not possible with the biological plan because although all follow the same format, each is unique. I have tried to describe that format, not prescribe actions. We must not try to impose still another adult prescription on that plan, which is how it gets wrecked in the first place.

Bonding is the issue, regardless of age. The parent who can start off with a new infant is lucky because by bonding to that infant they are bonding to the undifferentiated primary process. Learning to take our cues from the child and make a corresponding response means learning to heed and respond to the primary process within ourselves as well. A child can teach us an incredible amount if we are willing to learn, and because s/he is biologically geared to take his/her cues from us, s/he learns as we do.

Some specific steps are certainly apparent. Holding, with body molding, eye contact, smiling, and soothing sounds, is something all of us can use. Anything that blocks bonding should be avoided. Hospitals for delivery, bottles for feeding, cribs for sleeping, playpens and strollers for isolation, day-care centers for not caring, nursery schools for not nurturing, preschools—all create abandonment and weaken the bond. Surely, a parent would do everything possible to protect the child from premature literacy and be warned about television. To nurture the magical child is a full-time responsibility.

Surely the same holds for us adults who would reclaim our lives from anxiety's grip. Our lives, too, are filled with cues concerning real needs. The biological plan might go underground in this strange semantic reality of ours, but it is impossible for it to be extinguished. A full language system is found in both hemispheres of the child's brain, but later the right hemisphere goes mute. Although we are conditioned to orient to language feedback until it seems to fill the stage, the rest of the mind-brain goes right ahead as genetically planned. As my examples have shown, the primary process and the old brain's body-knowing continue right along. We adults face a signal-to-noise ratio problem. Our semantic reality, kept intact through our roof-brain chatter, makes an awful din, but we grow afraid of silence. We need to learn again to listen to our body and our primary process. They have their language, too, though it is not of the same nature as the propositional logic chattering in our heads.

The father who was suddenly moved to join his son in stopping the flow of blood had somehow broken through the noise level of his ordinary anxiety and followed the subtle signals of his body. A certain risk seems inherent in this kind of action, though, because it leads into unpredictable territory. Indeed, we have historically referred to this kind of nonordinary response as *left-handed thinking* because the right hemisphere, which runs the left hand, seems the repository for this kind of effect. Cultures have always represented this left hand as the sinister, dark, and evil largely because of its unpredictability. Had that father followed the predictable path of reaction, an entire chain of predictable forces would have been enacted: perhaps the sympathetic rescue squad and dramatic sirens wailing, sympathetic police and dramatic hospital emergency room, sympathetic doctors and nurses and maybe even the drama of the local news media and a human-interest story. Surely vast machinery would lie idle if left-hand thinking were to be employed habitually.

Our anxiety conditioning leads us to believe this left-hand process is tantamount to death itself, and our conditioning sets up buffers between this dark unknown and our ordinary awareness, which is sustained by verbal feedback and that which is right. Attuned to this noise, we lose our communication with the subtle power of the rest of our being. To become quiet and respond according to these subtle signals seems to be the equivalent of giving up our last defense. Yet, the moment we can drop such defenses, even for a brief time, and respond to our left hand, we shift matrix from anxiety to the primary process within.

A remarkable woman in her early thirties, formerly an actress, now working for a doctorate in psychology, related the following incident at a seminar.

As she was approaching her apartment in New York City late one evening, a car suddenly pulled up, and she was yanked into the front seat between two young men, a knife point immediately jabbing at her throat, all in the wink of an eye. The two young men immediately began babbling at her, their speech sporadic and half incoherent, that they were taking her out to New Jersey and were going to rape and kill her. They demanded that she tell them how it felt to be getting ready to die. It dawned on her that they meant it, that they were in a state of high agitation and had all the earmarks of intense fear and anger. They shook physically, the knife point at her throat jogging little stabs.

After an initial panic, realization of the futility of her position and a calm acceptance of her death swept over her. She replied to their frenzied questions calmly and earnestly. Now that she had accepted her death, her focus clarified and shifted. She became increasingly intrigued over the young men's fear and almost total lack of physical control. An odd maternal concern over them began to dominate her thoughts. She asked them about themselves, although they only insisted, like broken records, that she tell them what it felt like to be getting ready to die. She told them that she was sorry she had to die because she was young but that she understood perfectly well what the rape-kidnap laws were and realized why they would have to kill her. But what, she asked them, were they so afraid of? Why were they shaking so?

It was a strange conversation as they drove the thirty-odd miles out into a desolate, deserted part of the Jersey tidewater region. The men grew exasperated, confused, and more belligerent, all but pleading that she tell them how it felt to be getting ready to die. She prodded them with gentle, spontaneous, and utterly sincere questions about themselves and about why, knowing they had to do as they must do, they were so afraid. She assured them that all was well, that they did not have to be concerned on her account.

They arrived at a place that seemed familiar to them and in the dim light pointed out to her several mounds they claimed to be previous victims. Demanding that she tell them how it felt to be the next, they stripped her and threw her to the ground, both now whimpering and making strange noises. Looking up at the boy mounted over her, she dimly sensed a contorted and broken face. Compassion filled her anew, and she put her hands up, cradled his cheeks in her palms, and said quietly, "It's all right. You don't have to be afraid."

At this, the young man collapsed into a heap, overcome with great, wracking sobs, shaking uncontrollably in the spasm of wild grief. The other man sat pounding the ground and shouting, "What is it? What is it? What's gone wrong?" Then he, too, burst into the same strange, grief-stricken sobs.

It was some time before they quieted enough that she could speak to them and say quietly, "Boys, we may as well go home." Without a word, only their continued sobbing, they drove her back to the city. At the first subway, she suggested they let her out, which they did. She told us she had $300 in her purse, but they had given no thought to money. On impulse, she asked them would they lend her the money for the subway, which they did. She turned her back to them, started down the steps, heard them drive away, put her money in the turnstile, walked through, and fainted dead away. When she was questioned by the policeman who revived her, she replied, "If I told you, you'd never believe me."

What had happened here? The unbonded male rapes. He turns on the matrix in fear and rage to seize what was denied him and crush that matrix at the same time. But just as some autistic children seem most fearful of the physical nurturing they once so sorely needed, so these young men could not cope with freely given tenderness and compassion. The only state they could comprehend was a mirroring of their own isolation and terror. They pleaded with her to be terrified and reflect a madness they could understand. It was impossible, though, for them to act out their roles once she had accepted her death. She was then invulnerable, for how can you threaten a person who is already, in effect, dead? Anxiety arises from avoidance of the fact of our death; whereas muscular-mindedness arises from the ability to meet it. Accepting her death shifted her matrix. Like the aikido master, she walked through their rage untouched. She had inadvertently surrendered to the common ground between them, a continuum of possibility that works equally for all aspects of itself. She was then given the words to speak and the actions to take, just as the father of the bleeding child had been; and like that father, she gave the sanction of a safe space these young men had never known. For that brief space of time, they were bonded, their wounds also healed, and they wept.

Another story was related to us by a dear elderly woman. I can vouch for its authenticity in spite of its grade-C movie quality.

The year was 1903. She was nine years old, spending a year with her grandparents on a Kansas homestead. It was wild country back then, with lonely homesteads spread out over the land. The grandparents were Bible-belt fundamentalists, referring to the Lord with every breath in a kind of semantic reinforcement of their system of beliefs. They did not have locks on their doors, for instance, feeling that this would place their trust and faith outside the Lord.

One cold, rainy night, the grandfather, an itinerant preacher as well as farmer, was called away to sit with a dying member of his flock, and the little girl was allowed to sleep with her grandmother, a great treat. They heated the house with open-grate fireplaces, and the grandmother had banked the fire for the night (heaping ashes on top of a packed firebed to prevent rapid burning). It threw a soft pink glow over the bedroom. Some-time in the middle of the night, the little girl popped awake with a feeling of panic. Her grandmother was sitting up, and the little girl sat up immedi-ately, seeing, even as she opened her eyes and moved, a great, hulking figure of a man, rain dripping from his chin, poised over them, a large chunk of firewood in his hand, raised high. She felt a scream burbling up from her belly, but her grandmother quickly touched her, and a flood of calm swept her.

The grandmother was saying to the man, "I'm glad you found our house. You've come to the right place. The door was unlocked for you. You are welcomed here. It's a bad night to be out. You are cold, wet, and hungry. Take the firewood you have there, go in, and stir up the kitchen stove. Let me get a wrap on, and I will find you some dry clothes, fix you a good hot meal and a pallet behind the stove to sleep, where it's good and warm."

She said no more but calmly waited. A long pause ensued. Slowly the stick lowered, and the man said his only words the entire visit: "I won't hurt you."

He did as requested, and she did as promised. When he had been fed well and gone to his pallet in dry clothes, she returned to bed and fell immedi-ately to sleep. They awoke to find him gone. About ten o'clock that morning (and here the grade-C movie begins), they heard the baying of bloodhounds. A sherrif's posse charged into the yard in high excitement. Their night visitor, it appeared, had been the proverbial escaped homicidal maniac. He had stopped at their nearest neighbors' that very night, broken in, and systematically killed every member of the household, the grim condition of the home indicating a ghastly struggle. The sherrif had feared a duplicate of the disaster and was relieved to find the grandmother and child safe.

A reconstruction is not hard to make. The demon-ridden madman had escaped his captivity, plunged desparately through the cold night, spotted the farmhouse, broken into it. At sight of him, the family had panicked, no doubt screaming, rushing for guns, knives, hatchets. A general melee had ensued. His disorder of mind had been amply mirrored, amplified by their reacting energies. They had met his violence with their own and doubled the score.

He could not tolerate the house once the mayhem was over, seeing his madness reflecting in the carnage. So he plunged out in his terror, coming eventually to the grandmother's house. But then he entered a different environment. He met with unity. His madness found, not mirroring, but absorption, acceptance, and transformation. The primary process within him was then powered by the primary process in the grandmother, following her volitional decision, as primary process is designed to do when decision matches intent. She responded to the needs of the situation, and the needs were met—including hers and her grandchild's. It was impossible that the madman could have acted other than he did. It was not possible within her world for him to have been less than his true self. She freed him from his demon, at least for those fleeting hours.

Corny? Yes. But a pretty handy trick in case of trouble. The two cases cited cover, in fact, a good bit of our current locked-fortress urban, suburban, and now even rural dilemma and can apply equally to the most mundane family situations, although we revert to it only in dire extremes. In each case, the woman gave the men a safe space, a source of power to be more than their previous shackled selves, a source of possibility freed from the deadly fixations that held them. There was no justice in our usual social sense, no bringing of the bad guys to the gallows they so justly deserved. None of that. Nature has no justice in this sense. Her only justice is a unity in which all benefit.

These cases represent concrete operational thinking working as it should. As in walking the fire, the mind-brain takes in its information, operates on that information, and changes it, transforming the situation. But understand the profound difference between the examples given and the notion of "willing" someone to do something or outwitting an adversary by clever manipulation. Such domination, or trying to act on and forcibly change, would have brought disaster.

A friend said, "Ah, I get it. All of my life I have gone into every next event asking, in effect, What's in it for me? Now I see that what I must do is go into every event asking, What can I do for them?" And my friend had grievously missed the point. The great discovery is that we have nothing to give at all to anyone, anywhere. All we are designed to do is receive. Our hands are held out empty, not full of gifts for the less fortunate. I am a receiver, a perceiver, not the producer with largesse to dispense. I have nothing to give. Rather, I have sharp, specific needs from every situation. And so has each and every member of every situation. To deny ourselves is nonsense. And yet to act for ourselves is folly because we then try to direct our situation along the volitional lines of our either-or logic. The parts making up any situation regress infinitely out in every direction. Our intention must immediately clash with the counterintentions of others in every situation, each out to force the flow their way and make us react to suit their plans. All that can result from this is chaos, the usual cultural condition.

No, I bring nothing except my volitional ability to respond to the needs of the situation. To respond to the needs is simply to open, to say yes to the inner intent without attempting to understand, and then to just act as though. This play in the face of apparent hostility and problems is a kind of deep play, a play for very high stakes. This play keeps me alert. I know that I am not the producer, only the recipient, and that all I can do is play. But because of my willingness to play on the surface, the work underneath can then take place. So what I play, what I pretend, is that the work *is* taking place, even though I cannot know that for sure ahead of time or know how it will unfold. I pretend as though and find, to my delight and continual surprise, that the world out there bends to my desire. And what is my desire? That as I respond to the needs of the situation, those needs will be met. I do not have to try to figure the correct choices among the myriads of possibilities; I have only to say yes to my intent. Then the right words and actions are given to me.

God works, and man plays—or that is the way the scheme is set up and meant to be. I like it that way. As soon as I try to do all the work, I have tried to be God, and I mess everything up. The harder I play, the harder God works. Sometimes we get caught up in a spinning around of this work-play. Sometimes everything catches fire in this work-play spiral, a spiral of fire such as Blaise Pascal experienced and scrawled about on that piece of paper one marvelous night: "Fire! Fire!" he wrote, "not the god of philosophy, but the God of Abraham, of Isaac, and of Jacob." He had fallen into play, was never the same again, and carried his scrawled response in the lining of his coat, next to his heart, all his life.

Perhaps this is not a very detailed prescription, but it will meet the needs of any child entrusted to us—the offspring we begot or will beget, conceived or will conceive, and this child eternally begotten in ourselves.

Notes

Chapter 1. *Promise Given: Magnificent Heritage*
1. See Thomas Lewis, *The Lives of a Cell.*
2. In response to psychologists' complaint that "it is inconceivable that so much information could be built into a brain without interaction between the behavior and the environment," Blurton Jones states: "Many zoologists have become resigned to finding natural selection capable of producing almost any achievement." See Jones, *Ethological Studies of Child Behavior,* p. 16.
3. In a recent address, Karl Pribram elaborated on his theory of the brain as a hologram and suggested that the earth, too, is a hologram. The individual microcosmic hologram thus reflects the macrocosmic one, an idea held and practiced in the East. We enter into a realm of operational thinking by acting back into the macrocosmic hologram. See Pribram, *Language of the Brain,* chapter 8.
4. See Greenough, *The Nature and Nurture of Behavior.*
5. See Jerome Bruner, *The Relevance of Education,* p. 53. Bruner speaks for the current notion that prolonged childhood is necessary so that the culture's cumulative knowledge might be taught the child. Hans G. Furth does not suit a curricula for the marketplace so well but is far more accurate. A few lines from Furth are pertinent here: "The development of intelligence is the result not of some outside factor but of an internal regulating force that is not solely or primarily dependent on the objects with which the intellect is in contact." See Furth, *Piaget for Teachers,* p. 5. "Intelligence has its own laws of internal growth . . . its successive acquisitions are not merely drawn by cumulative

additions from the child's physical or social environment." See Furth, *Piaget and Knowledge,* p. 222. Bruner (on p. 57 of *The Relevance of Education*) considers the five great humanizing forces to be tool making, language, society, management of childhood, and the compulsion to explain. We build tools in a direct ratio to our loss of personal power, however; the impulse toward language is genetically coded and is used for wider capacities than Bruner sees; we have, not a society, but a legally imposed culture based on semantic idea systems rather than interacting relationships; we manage childhood as we manage our politics, industries, and/or any semantic idea system and thoroughly fail to nurture the child's intelligence; and we start compulsively explaining as we lose our power to act. On page 120 of the same work, Bruner clarifies the issue at stake by quoting Washburn: "Without culture and tools man would be among the ecologically unimportant primates." This shallow talk ignores that man has been on this earth for 3 million years or more and that you cannot have a brain system that does not function, at least as partially as ours now does, in accord with that brain's structure. Evidence is ample that superior civilizations have risen and fallen regularly over the millennia. A society of people fully functioning in the three modes of intelligence we have within us would need no tools and leave no artifacts. Hans Furth's twenty-five years of work with congenitally deaf children (who have *no* access to any linguistic system) shows that these children nevertheless develop intelligence and logic on a slow, orderly unfolding as outlined by Piaget. These people learn to function in an essentially hostile environment, against extreme odds, and without semantic process, the key tool our reality system is built around.

When Bruner states (on page 122 of *The Relevance of Education*) that any subject can be taught at any age in some form, he states a disastrous half-truth. The issue is not *can* we so engineer the emerging mind. Rather, it is what is appropriate to the needs of the child at a particular stage. We speak of a "blind technology," but that technology is nothing but the highest products of our education system, the minds successfully managed and taught according to this notion of earlier and earlier academic learning. A blind technology raping the earth means blind minds trained to run that system.

Chapter 2. Matrix Shifts: Known to Unknown

1. Death is the ultimate abstraction out of concreteness, toward which the system is oriented. Mind is never the content of experience; but rather, it is the ability to interact gained through that experience. Nature never brings about a matrix shift without providing ample bonding, or establishing points of similarity with the next matrix, because that would be self-defeating. Bonding is thus the essence of intellectual growth. Maturation should automatically be a bonding with the matrix that follows physical death.

Chapter 4. Stress and Learning

1. I picked up the term *sensory sampling* from Zipf. He also called it the *peephole effect.* See George Kingsley Zipf, *The Psycho Biology of Language,* p. 167.
2. Conceptual brain patterning, according to E. Roy John ("How the Brain Works —A New Theory"), takes place through synchronous rhythmic patterns of cell activity, a "statistical operation" among large numbers of cells, often quite distant from each other. A single cell contributes to the average behavior of a

large group of cells, and the pattern of all gives us perception and thought. Cells fire continously and sporadically. Random, unpatterned activity creates "noise" as opposed to the rhythmic patterns giving signals. Any cell may contribute to any pattern of rhythms, and all parts of the brain seem to take part in all activities. From Epstein's work, we find that new cell connections, preparing for new learning, seem to take place in large spurts on a periodic basis about every four years (during development). John finds that new learning does not bring about new cell connections; rather, cells in many parts of the brain learn a new rhythm of firing corresponding to the learning.

3. A young M.D. acquaintance of mine told of making this study in graduate school by placing live rat brain cells on a microscopic slide, adding ACTH, and watching almost instant growth of new connecting links spring up.

4. Our ordinary left-hemisphere logic operates on a two-pronged basis: yes-no, either-or, an elaboration of an ativistic flight-fight differentiation of logic. Through anxiety, we get locked into this binary system and lose our other forms of logic, such as that of primary processing, where the law of the excluded middle of our Western either-or does not hold. Solving mathematical problems gives a good indication of this linear, competent, and useful either-or logic. When you solve a math problem, the right answer suddenly occurs to you. Studies show that shortly after, as a kind of shadow effect, the opposite, or wrong, answer also forms. Logical feedback presents both its either and its or. We can build technology with either-or, but we cannot heal disease, walk fire, or develop personal power or creativity thereby.

Chapter 5. New Demonology: Exorcising Nature

1. Ashley Montagu, recognizing the critical importance of skin stimulus in the newborn, suggested that the human's prolonged labor is necessary to provide this vital stimulus. This would be a good observation if that prolonged labor were natural and if the mother's ignoring of or isolation from the newborn were natural, but none of this is the case. See Montagu, *Touching*.

Chapter 6. Time Bomb: In the Delivery Room

1. I will hazard the hypothesis that the interaction is between the preprogrammed old-brain cells, carrying the 3-billion-year heritage, and the new-brain cells that will act as the computer-creator, acting on and out of this heritage. The interaction taking place may well be to set up a predisposition in those new-brain cells to accept, over a range of nearly infinite flexibility, that thrust coded into the old-brain cells as a general intent. Furthermore, this same mixing and interacting of the different cell types would provide the predisposition toward the brain functioning as a hologram; that is, any cell would take part in the total brain activity while yet specializing, and so be able, if necessary, to function as the whole.

2. In 1966, T. G. R. Bower, working with infants from two weeks of age up, found they would respond to visual tests provided an interesting-enough reward was offered, that reward proving to be peekaboo administered by a woman assistant when the infant gave a correct response. Bower reported: "Infants between two and twenty weeks old seem to find this event highly reinforcing and will respond for 20 minutes at a time to make it [peekaboo] occur. . . . even infants as young as two weeks old can give 400 such responses with no apparent

fatigue." See Bower, "The Visual World of the Infant." (Bear this in mind when we discuss play.)

In 1967, Hanus Papousek described getting infants hungry to see if food as a stimulus would enhance learning response. (It works with rats.) He set up listening experiments in which, if the infant correctly solved the problem and activated the proper switch (by turning their head), they were rewarded with a feeding nipple. A wrong solution response brought a nonfeeding nipple. Thus, theoretically, the hungrier they were, the more attentive they would be. Papousek has lovely photographs of infants in the third month "smiling when they have learned to predict the side on which a feeding nipple will appear on the basis of a signal tone preceding it." Now, the interesting thing was, the infants were smiling at having successfully analyzed and responded to the complex of signals, not at gaining the food. For no matter that they were hungry, they turned down actually nursing at the nipple, instead, each time turning eagerly back to the researcher with a beaming smile of delight over their success, wanting to play again. The intrinsic reward of *play* proved greater than the extrinsic reward of food. See Papousek, "Experimental Studies of Appetitional Behavior in Human Newborns and Infants."

In 1970, Kalnins reported on infant visual response. He noticed that infants will automatically suck when a nipple is put in their mouth, so he rigged up an electronic nipple that registered the number of sucks per minute. Then he placed the infant, with this electronic nipple, in front of a movie screen on which a film was shown out of focus. If the infant hit a certain prescribed fast rate of sucking (statistically probable), that prescribed rate would bring the movie into focus. Thus, if the infant could distinguish between a focused and unfocused flat-screen projection, perhaps they would prefer the focused variety, connect the sucking rate with the visual response, and work to maintain the focus. A further complication lies in an early infant being unable to suck and focus at the same time; either entrainment absorbs the total brain attention. Nevertheless, the infants easily caught on and further established a delicate balance between establishing the necessary focus by proper fast sucking, then focusing to enjoy the show. As the machinery then registered the lack of sucking and phased out the focus, the wily infant resumed sucking to reinstate focus, hitting a neat balance that kept maximum focus with minimum attention to sucking. Once the infants had caught on to this, the researchers changed the rate of sucking necessary to maintain focus, right in the middle of the experiment. It took the average infant an average of four seconds to catch on to the shift and reestablish a new rate of sucking. A reversal shift was then employed. Once the game was well established, the infant was placed before a screen with the movie already in focus. Immediately, they fell into the proper rhythmic pattern of suck-focus to enjoy the show. This time, however, sucking blurred the picture. It took the average infant an average of eight seconds to catch on to this complete reversal and adopt to the new pattern.

3. Infant synchrony with speech has been authenticated by subsequent studies. Marshall Klaus, in a lecture-demonstration in San Francisco (1976) showed film of a mother repeating a phrase to her highly active new infant. When the

film was run in slow motion, the infant's movements were seen to be identical with each repetition, as though they were a dance step to the words.

4. Suzanne Arms describes how this highly unnatural and disruptive position got started in the West. Louis XIV was sexually aroused by watching his mistresses bear his young. Unable to see well enough because of the crouch or squat position (almost universally employed) he had his attendants make the poor women lie on their backs. The doctors emulated this exalted example, and it became the rage, the popular thing to do. Then it became the custom and thus unquestioned. Long and difficult labors, making nurturing afterward almost impossible, thus began the vicious double bind.

5. A fine M.D. friend of mine, an ophthalmologist, was upset by my seminar statements from Windle and others that premature umbilical severing took place in a majority of all medical births. He pointed out that every obstetrical text emphasized leaving the cord strictly alone until all activity in it ceased. He could not believe doctors had abandoned such a commonplace and obvious necessity. A young doctor, some three years out of medical school, told me, however, that in his internship in a large eastern hospital, he had delivered ten babies under supervision and that he had been *instructed* not only to cut the cord immediately that it was available but also then to jerk the cord to dislodge the placenta—the quicker to get the delivery room cleared. Two obstetrical nurses testified that my evidence was, if anything, understated, that the actual situation was far more grim.

6. M. P. M. Richards reports on the many ways Pethilorfan, the most widely used drug in Britain, affects both mother and newborn and how the newborn's physical responses (first breathing and so forth) are far more retarded and still very much so *weeks* later. More seriously, Richards's studies showed how mother-infant relations were dramatically altered by the drugged state of each, patterns of relationship never again altered, but setting the stage for the entire childhood period. See Blurton N. Jones, *Ethological Studies of Child Behavior,* chapter 7.

7. See Suzanne Arms, *Immaculate Deception.*

Chapter 7.   Breaking the Bond: Our End Is in Our Beginning; Our Beginning Is Our End

1. Jean MacKellar's is in the form of a personal communication.

2. See Blurton N. Jones, *Ethological Studies of Child Behavior,* chapter 11, pp. 305–328.

3. Data have been gathering since the 1940s showing specific harm to infants and to mother-infant relations. Montagu gives clear evidence of this in *Prenatal Influences.*

4. John Ott is the originator of time-lapse photography and is now considered the world's foremost authority on the effects of light on living things. His documentary film clearly shows the harmful effects of fluorescence, particularly the pink spectrum, its role in cancer, leukemia, and hyperactivity in children. More and more new schools are being built without windows (children look out of them in longing for the world they were meant to be in) and lighted with fluorescence.

5. Back in 1924, Otto Rank, following Freud's nonsense, wrote of life in the womb being such perfect bliss and birth from it such trauma that we spend our lives

looking for a womb substitute or return to the womb. Of course, the organism is built for stress-relaxation cycles of growth, and Freud's whole notion of the "oceanic bliss" of the womb as a source of religion and so on, as well as his notion that stress causes anxiety and that the organism tries to avoid stress, is typical nonsense.

6. The shock of abandonment is the issue we face. We take abandoning the infant for granted. The television commercial shows the young mothers outside the glass-walled nursery, pointing sweetly to their abandoned infants while sweet music plays and sweet voices sell sweetly perfumed disposable diapers.

Chapter 8.   Concept: Do You See?

1. I use right-left hemisphere theory as a model, a working example of how functions might take place. The function is the fact; the model is simply the attempt to represent the function in a graphic way. For example, we speak of the brain as a "computer" and can then look at our machines that compute and find a model for a function. But to equate the model and the function as a theory is risky.

Chapter 10.   Establishing the Matrix

1. The model mother is based on conversations with new mothers around the country and on descriptions found in the works of LeBoyer, Geber, Ainsworth, Klaus and others. At a seminar, a young Englishwoman with two healthy, bright youngsters in tow described both deliveries at home, by herself. She locked the door to assure privacy, wanting this experience completely to herself, and she knew ecstacy both times.

2. Sensing infants in utero is vital and is *not* romantic hypothesis. But it is difficult in surroundings of noise, confusion, hostility, anxiety. The signal-to-noise ratio is a problem, as it is with all primary processing, but the meditative or natural state opens one to natural communications.

3. Marshall Klaus spoke of the mother as having a kind of "glue" on her head during the first hour after birth that is designed to seal that new infant right into her. The presence of other people tends to siphon off this magnetic energy. Privacy is critical.

4. The warm bath is certainly optional but not to be discounted. Establishing points of similarity between new and old matrices is the issue, but the cues must be taken from the infant, any meaningless ritual must be avoided.

5. Nursing at birth immediately acts on the mother's abdominal muscles, pulling the uterus back into shape and retoning the whole area.

6. A sling for carrying should be part of mother's garment, allowing the naked infant to remain in contact with her bare breasts. Critical body-heat problems are thereby avoided, and the infant can feed continuously, retain eye contact with the mother, and receive much needed continual human skin stimulus. In turn, the mother is in proximity to sense the infant's general state and respond appropriately. Furthermore, she is free to pursue her normal affairs.

Chapter 11.   World As It Is

1. Ability is intelligence, not information recall. The brain does not process ability by memory checks against previous encounters; it does so by checking the abilities achieved through previous interactions. A weight lifter's muscles build through his training, but his body does not check back over all previous lifts

in order to activate the muscles. Ability is a condition, a capacity independent of any process of arrival to that condition. Most of what the young learn in school is obsolete by the time they graduate. Thus, the information is worthless. It does not give the ability to interact with greater expanses of experience; rather, it gives the ability to interact with a highly specific, limited, and self-verifying type of closed semantic system. This is not intelligence in any full sense.

Chapter 12. Filling in the Details

1. Cross-culturally, children seem to see the world in the same way until after age seven. The drawings of a four-year-old in Kansas are nearly identical to those of a four-year-old in Timbuctoo. After age seven, cultural differences begin to show. See Rhoda Kellog, *Analyzing Children's Art*.

2. Piaget claimed what we see is no indication of what is necessarily there. In his article "The Resources of Binocular Perception in the Visual System," John Ross explored this "editorial" quality of perception, describing it as "unconscious interpretation of visual data," in which the brain decides what it will see. Visual "records" are consulted before anything is seen, so that vision is a "critical faculty capable of making decisions and of rejecting information, apparently on esthetic grounds." Furthermore, we apparently idealize what we see. The visual system may have a program, an arrangement for perceiving shapes in time and space. "What we see is an interpretation." "We adopt a perceptual attitude in order to comprehend the world" (or, I would suggest, in order to make the world conform to our semantic system).

3. Brain activity is virtually ceaseless. This conceptual activity will produce percepts by its own actions if perceptual stimuli are unavailable to the senses. Sensory isolation, in which no information comes in, prompts this conceptual system to produce its own sensory stimuli. The perceived experience is the same in either case; a percept is a percept. Bear this in mind when I talk about creating reality experience or shared creations of reality.

4. Richard Curtis, of St. George Homes in Berkeley, California, related a similar experience with a teen-age schizophrenic patient. She asked him to make the terrible demons riding and nagging her leave her alone, and he agreed with her, joined with her in meeting those demons and telling them to go way. They did. See Charles Tart, *Altered States of Consciousness*, and Kilton Stewart's account of a similar technique employed by the Senoi.

Chapter 13. Division of Labor: Birthing a Self

1. Observations by Lee Sannella, M.D., in *Psychosis or Transcendence?* led to this whole synthesis.

2. See Walter Stace, *The Teachings of the Mystics*.

3. Cannon, in *The Wisdom of the Body*, observed that our physical-chemical "milieu intérieur" remained constant in the variable "milieu extérieur." George Zipf once noted: "The preservation of homeostasis is not the goal of the organism . . . rather [it is] an economical device for survival."

Chapter 14. Primary Perceptions: Bonding with the Earth

1. I have only news clippings and personal reports on Jampolsky's work.

2. See James Peterson, *Some Profiles of Non-ordinary Perception of Children*.

3. See *National Geographic*, June 1976.

4. See Mathew Manning, *The Link*, for Dr. Whitton's comments.

5. See Lee Sannella, *Psychosis or Transcendence?;* see also Paramahansa Yoga-nanda, *Autobiography of a Yogi,* for yogi views. David Bressler, UCLA, reports ancient Chinese acupuncture knowledge of energy flows.

6. Farley Mowatt wrote *Never Cry Wolf* as a result of a long-term study of wolves undertaken for the Canadian government.

7. See Blurton N. Jones, *Ethological Studies of Child Behavior,* chapter 8.

8. I got this from Harry Stack Sullivan, *The Interpersonal Theory of Psychiatry.*

9. See Peterson, *Some Profiles of Non-ordinary Perception of Children.*

Chapter 15.   Play: In the Service of Survival

1. See Mihaly Csikszentmihalyi, "Play and Intrinsic Rewards," for a most impressive study (possibly attainable from Association for Humanistic Psychology, 325 Ninth Street, San Francisco, Calif. 94730).

Chapter 16.   Dancing through the Crack: Operational Thinking

1. Acquaintances of mine spent a short time in Bali a couple of years ago making movies of nonordinary cultural practices. They found no dancing over coals, as they did on Fiji and other islands. Belo's study was made a number of years ago, and because the phenomena fit the stage unfolding at seven, I have accepted her reports (she was there a long time). See Jane Belo, *Trance in Bali.*

2. See Edmund Carpenter, *Oh, What a Blow That Phantom Gave Me.*

3. Stopping bleeding has a long history; yoga adepts can do this, and it can be done through hypnosis. Ainslee Meares, an Australian physician, has written extensively on bloodless surgery; see Meares, *A System of Medical Hypnosis.*

4. See my book, *The Crack in the Cosmic Egg,* chapter 6, for a description.

Chapter 17.   The Two-Way Flow: Assimilation-Accommodation

1. See Mathew Manning, *The Link.*

Chapter 18.   Toward Autonomy: Splitting the Brain

1. See Sylvia Anthony, *The Child's Discovery of Death,* for the best study I have found (made in England during World War II); Adah Maurer, "Maturation of Concepts of Death," is the next best; Gregory Rochlin, "Fears of Death and Religious Beliefs," is very poor, out to validate psychoanalytic thought, not to explore what a child thinks.

2. See Joseph Chilton Pearce, *The Crack in the Cosmic Egg.*

3. See Robert Ornstein, *The Nature of Human Consciousness* and *The Psychology of Consciousness.*

4. Michael Gazzaniga wondered why the brain would make its most elaborate and difficult construction, language, in both hemispheres, as found in the child, only to deconstruct this construction in the right hemisphere somewhere before age twelve. He observed that nowhere else in nature do we find such a lapse of economy. I have given at least part of the answer: What should have been a functional separation for an interacting relationship becomes, through anxiety conditioning, a schism, the balance imbalanced. Certainly, logical maturation and the growth of abstract thinking require a separation of word from thing and of self from world, but in the same sense as separation of infant from the womb—for a greater relationship, not isolation and abandonment.

5. Internalizing speech is one of logic's great tools for abstract thinking, as Bruner explores so well. What nature did not intend was internal speech as a compulsive feedback mechanism to sustain a nonreal semantic system.

6. See Joseph Chilton Pearce, *Exploring the Crack in the Cosmic Egg,* for a fairly good description of roof-brain chatter. Before nine or ten, the child's mind is quiet; language feedback systems are not yet employed as semantic stabilizers because the semantic-reality system is not yet completely dominant.

Chapter 19. The Cycle of Creative Competence

1. Children who read spontaneously or learn to read very early have been read to extensively by parents and in fantasy-type reading. The child, whose fantasy needs are thus being met (storytelling would be far better) catches on to the system and learns to read in order to enter freely that world of inner space. Furth claims schoolchildren doing well in early reading generally do so to maintain sanction bonding with parents and teachers, moving against the natural flow of the body system to avoid abandonment by his superiors. See Furth, *Piaget and Knowledge* and *Piaget for Teachers.* There is an additional note on the possible effects of premature literacy and its split of biological function: 100 years ago Scandinavian women began menstruation at an average age of seventeen. Today, after a century of premature literacy, that age is fourteen. Mediterranean women began menstruation at an average age of fourteen; today, its eleven. Early in this century, Rudolph Steiner claimed that premature academic learning stepped up genital sexuality, a subject needing thorough research.

Chapter 20. *Thinking about Thinking: Formal Operations*

1. See Edmund Carpenter, *Eskimo Realities.*

2. I have simplified Piaget's detailed studies on this phenomenon.

3. See Jerome Bruner, *The Relevance of Education,* p. 27.

4. See Marilyn Ferguson, *The Brain Revolution,* and O.W. Markley, "Suggestology."

Chapter 21. Journey into the Mind: Creative Reality

1. See Joseph Chilton Pearce, *The Crack in the Cosmic Egg,* for a discussion of Kekule.

2. See Ann Faraday, *The Dream Game,* and Charles Tart, *Altered States of Consciousness.*

3. See Tart, *Altered States of Consciousness.*

Bibliography

To keep this work readable and within bounds, I have avoided direct reference to supportive research, with some exceptions. My use of this material has been general and synthetic. Much of this material was kindly sent by people attending my seminars, and all of it proved apropos and helpful. But I can hardly say that I agree with the intent, attitude, or conclusions of the research in all cases.

Aaron, Michael. "The World of the Brain." *Harper's Magazine,* Wraparound, December 1975.

Ainsworth, Mary D. *Deprivation of Maternal Care: A Reassessment of Its Effects.* Public Health Papers no. 14, pp. 97–165. Geneva: World Health Organization.

————. *Infancy in Uganda.* Baltimore: Johns Hopkins University Press, 1967.

————. "Patterns of Attachment Behavior Shown by the Infant in Interaction with His Mother." *Merril-Palmer Quarterly* 10 (1964): 51–58.

Almy, M. *Young Children's Thinking: Studies of Some Aspects of Piaget's Theory.* New York: Teachers College Press, 1966.

Anthony, Sylvia. *The Child's Discovery of Death: A Study in Child Psychology.* London: Kegan Paul, Trench, 1940.

Arms, Suzanne. *Immaculate Deception: A New Look at Women and Childbirth in America.* Boston: Houghton Mifflin Company, 1975.

Bateson, Gregory. *Steps to an Ecology of Mind.* New York: Ballantine Books, 1972.

Beadle, Muriel. *A Child's Mind: How Children Learn During the Critical Years from Birth to Age Five.* New York: Doubleday & Company, 1970.

Beck, Joan. *How to Raise a Brighter Child: The Case for Early Learning.* New York: Pocket Books, 1975.

Becker, Ernest. *The Denial of Death.* New York: The Free Press, 1973.

————. *The Revolution in Psychiatry: The New Understanding of Man.* New York: The Free Press, 1974.

Belo, Jane. *Trance in Bali.* New York: Columbia University Press, 1960.

Bengeldorf, Irving S. "Neural Mechanisms of Learning and Memory: Preliminary Report." *Department of Health, Education, and Welfare Bulletin,* August 1975.

Bernard, J., and Sontag, L. "Fetal Reactions to Sound." *Journal of Genetic Psychology* 70 (1947): 209–210.

Bohm, David. *Causality and Chance in Modern Physics.* Princeton, N.J.: Van Nostrand, 1957.

————. "Reality and Knowledge Considered as Process." *The Academy,* February 1975.

Bower, T. G. R. "The Visual World of the Infant." *Scientific American,* December 1966.

Bowlby, John. "The Child's Tie to His Mother: Attachment Behavior." In *Attachment.* New York: Basic Books, 1969.

————. "Maternal Care and Mental Health." Monograph Series no. 2, p. 5–10. Geneva: World Health Organization, 1951.

————. "Processes of Mourning." *International Journal of Psychoanalysis* 42 (1961): 317–334.

————. "Separation Anxiety." *International Journal of Psychoanalysis* 41: (1960) 89–113.

Brody, Sylvia, and Axelrod, S. *Anxiety and Ego Formation in Infancy.* New York: International Universities Press, 1970.

Bruner, Jerome. *Beyond the Information Given: Studies in the Psychology of Knowing.* New York: W. W. Norton & Company, 1973.

————. *On Knowing: Essays for the Left Hand.* Cambridge, Mass.: Harvard University Press, Belknap Press, 1962.

————. "Processes of Growth in Infancy." In *Stimulation in Early Infancy,* edited by A. Ambrose. London: Academic Press 1969.

————. *The Relevance of Education.* New York: W. W. Norton & Company, 1971.

Bruner, J., et al., *A Study of Thinking.* New York: Science Editions, 1962.

Burgers, J. M., "Causality and Anticipation." *Science,* 18 July 1975, pp. 194–198.

Burke, Frederick. "Two Orders of Learning." *Pedagogical Seminary,* September 1902. Reprint *Manas,* 18 February 1976.

Cannon, W. B. *The Wisdom of the Body.* New York: W. W. Norton & Company, 1939.

Carpenter, Edmund. *Eskimo Realities.* New York: Holt, Rinehart and Winston, 1973.

————. *Oh, What a Blow That Phantom Gave Me!* New York: Bantam Books, 1973.

Cassierer, Ernst. *Language and Myth.* New York: Harper & Row, Publishers, 1946.

Cheek, David. "Maladjustments May Be Results of Birth Events." *Brain-Mind Bulletin* 1, no. 7 (February 16, 1976): 1.

Chomsky, Noam. "Recent Contributions to the Theory of Innate Ideas." *Synthese* 17 (1967).

Condon, W., and Sander, Louis. "Neonate Movement Is Synchronized with Adult Speech: Interactional Participation and Language Acquisition." *Science,* 11 January 1974, pp. 99–101.

Connolly, Kevin, and Bruner, J., eds. *The Growth of Competence.* New York: Academic Press, 1974.

Cooper, David. *The Death of the Family.* New York: Random House, Vintage Books, 1971.

Csikszentmihalyi, Mihaly. "Play and Intrinsic Rewards." *Journal of Humanistic Psychology* 13, no. 3 (Summer 1975).

Curtis, Richard. "Aikido: The Way of Spiritual Harmony." Paper prepared for the faculty of St. George Homes, Berkeley, Calif.

Ehrenwald, Jan. "Brain Model for Processing Psychic Events." *Journal of Nervous and Mental Diseases,* as reported in *Brain-Mind Bulletin* 1, no. 6 (March 1, 1976):

Epstein, Herman T. "Phrenoblysis: Special Brain and Mind Growth Periods. I. Human Brain and Skull Development. II. Human Mental Development." In *Developmental Psychobiology,* New York: John Wiley & Sons, 1974.

Fantz, Robert L. "The Origin of Form Perception." *Scientific American,* May 1961, pp. 66–72.

————. "Pattern Vision in Young Infants." *Psychological Review* 8 (1958): 43–47.

Faraday, Ann. *The Dream Game.* New York: Harper & Row, Publishers, 1974.

Farnsworth, Pilar. "Reach Out for the Hours After Birth." *East West Journal* 5, no. 3 (March 1975).

Feinberg, Leonard. "Firewalking in Ceylon." *Atlantic Monthly,* May 1959.

Ferguson, Marilyn. *The Brain Revolution.* New York: Bantam Books, 1973.

Fisher, Charles, et al. "A Psychophysiological Study of Nightmares and Night Terrors." *Journal of Nervous and Mental Disease* 187, no. 2.

Flavell, John H. *The Developmental Psychology of Jean Piaget.* New York: D. Van Nostrand Company, 1963.

Fodor, J. A., et al. "Speech Discrimination in Infants." *Perception and Psychophysics* 18, no. 2 (1975): 74–78.

Foulkes, David. "Longitudinal Studies of Dreams in Children." In *Dreaming Dynamics,* edited by Masserman. Grune & Stratton, 1971.

Furth, Hans G. *Deafness and Learning.* New York: Wadsworth Publishing Co., 1973.

————. *Piaget and Knowledge.* Englewood Cliffs, N.J.: Prentice-Hall, 1969.

————. *Piaget for Teachers.* Englewood Cliffs, N.J.: Prentice-Hall, 1970.

————. *Thinking without Language.* New York: The Free Press, 1966.

Gardner, Lytt I. "Deprivation Dwarfism." *Scientific American,* July 1972, pp. 76–82.

Geber, Marcelle. "The Psycho-Motor Development of African Children in the First Year and the Influence of Maternal Behavior." *Journal of Social Psychology,* no. 47 (1958): 185–95.

Gilder, George F. *Naked Nomads.* New York: Quadrangle, The New York Times Book Co., 1974.

Ginott, Haim. *Between Parent and Child.* New York: Macmillan, 1965.

————. *Between Parent and Teenager.* New York: Macmillan, 1969.

Globus, Gordon G. "Unexpected Symmetries in the 'World Knot.' Apparently Disparate Monist and Dualist Views on Mind and Matter Are Held to Be Symmetric." *Science,* 15 June 1973, pp. 1129–1130.

Gordon, T. *P.E.T.: Parent Effectiveness Training.* Peter H. Wyden/Publisher, 1970.

Gray, P. H. "Imprinting in Infants." *Journal of Psychology* 46 (1958): 155–166.

Greenfield and Tronic. "Curriculum for the Day Care Center at Boston's Bromley-

Heath." In *The Relevance of Education,* Jerome Bruner. New York: W. W. Norton & Company, 1971.

Gregory, R. E. *Eye and Brain:* The Psychology of Seeing. New York: McGraw-Hill Book Company, 1966.

Harlow, Harry F. "Love in Infant Monkeys." *Scientific American,* June 1959, pp. 68–74.

Harlow, Harry, and Harlow, Margaret. "Social Deprivation in Monkeys." *Scientific American,* November 1962, pp. 136–146.

Harwood, A. C. *The Way of a Child: An Introduction to the Work of Rudolph Steiner for Children.* London: Rudolph Steiner Press, 1940.

Hess, Robert D., and Shipman, Virginia. "Early Experience and the Socialization of the Cognitive Modes in Children." *Child Development,* no. 36 (1965): 869–886.

Hilgard, Ernst. "Hypnosis Is No Mirage." *Psychology Today,* November 1974, pp. 120–128.

———. *Hypnotic Susceptibility.* New York: Harcourt Brace Jovanovich, 1965.

———. "Two Separate Cognitive Systems." *Brain-Mind Bulletin* 1, no. 9 (March 15, 1976).

Holt, John. *Instead of Education: Ways to Help People Do Things Better.* New York: E. P. Dutton, 1976.

Illich, Ivan. *Medical Nemesis.* New York: Pantheon Books, 1976.

John, E. Roy. "How the Brain Works—A New Theory." *Psychology Today,* May 1976, pp. 48–52.

Jones, Blurton N. *Ethological Studies of Child Behavior.* New York: Cambridge University Press, 1972.

Josephson, Brian. "Possible Connections between Psychic Phenomena and Quantum Mechanics." *The Academy* 14, no. 4 (December 1975).

Kaufman, C., and Rosenbloom, L. "Depression in Infant Monkeys." *Science,* 24 February 1967, pp. 1030–1031.

Kellog, Rhoda. *Analyzing Children's Art.* New York: National Press Books, 1969.

Kessen, W., ed. *Childhood in China.* New Haven: Yale University Press, 1975.

Klaus, Marshall, et al. "Human Maternal Behavior at the First Contact with Her Young." *Pediatrics* 46, no. 2 (August 1970): 187–192.

———. "Maternal Attachment: Importance of the First Post-Partum Days." *New England Journal of Medicine,* 286, no. 9 (March 2, 1972): 460–463.

Koestler, Leon. *The Act of Creation.* New York: Macmillan, 1964.

Lake, Alice. "New Babies Are Smarter Than You Think." *Woman's Day,* June 1976.

LeBoyer, Frederick *Birth without Violence.* New York: Alfred A. Knopf, 1974.

Levine, Seymour. "Stimulation in Infancy." *Scientific American,* May 1960, pp. 80–86.

Lewis, Thomas. *The Lives of a Cell.* New York: Viking Press, 1974.

Lowry, Lawrence. "Environmental Influences on Measures of Intelligence." Department of Education, University of California, Berkeley.

———. "First-Borns with Siblings vs. First-Borns without Siblings: A Sex Difference in Mental Test Performance." Department of Education, University of California, Berkeley.

Luria, Alexander R. *The Role of Speech in Normal and Abnormal Behavior.* New York: Liveright, 1961.

MacKellar, Jean. *Rape: The Bait and the Trap.* New York: Crown Publishers, 1975.

Manning, Matthew. *The Link.* London: Van Duren Press, 1975.

Markley, O. W. "Suggestology." Report for staff members, C. F. Kettering Foundation, Stanford Research Institute, Center for the Study of Social Policy, Menlo Park, Calif.

Massie, Henry. "The Early Natural History of Childhood Psychosis." *Journal of American Academy of Child Psychology,* in press.

———. "Patterns of Mother-Infant Behavior and Subsequent Childhood Psychosis: A Research and Case Report." Mt. Zion Hospital and Medical Center, San Francisco, 1975.

Maurer, Adah. "Maturation of Concepts of Death." *British Journal of Medical Psychology* (1966): 35.

Meares, Ainslie. *A System of Medical Hypnosis.* New York: Julian Press, 1961.

Mitchell, Gary. "What Monkeys Can Tell Us about Human Violence." *The Futurist,* April 1975.

Monroe, Robert. *Journeys Out of the Body.* New York: Doubleday & Company, 1973.

Montagu, Ashley. *Life before Birth.* New York: New American Library, 1964.

———. *The Natural Superiority of Women.* New York: Macmillan, 1968.

———. *Prenatal Influences.* Springfield, Ill.: Charles C. Thomas, Publisher, 1962.

———. *Touching: The Human Significance of the Skin.* New York: Columbia University Press, 1971.

Nakaoka, Toshiya. "Parapsychological Argument in Japan." *Bulletin, Japanese ESP Society,* 1975.

Ornstein, Robert. *The Nature of Human Consciousness.* New York: Viking Press, 1973.

———. *The Psychology of Consciousness.* San Francisco: Miller Freeman Publications, 1971.

Ostrander, S., and Schroder, L. *Psychic Discoveries behind the Iron Curtain.* New York: Bantam Books, 1971.

Panati, Charles, ed. *Geller Papers.* Boston: Houghton Mifflin Company, 1976.

Papousek, Hanus. "Experimental Studies of Appetitional Behavior in Human Newborns and Infants." In *Early Behavior,* edited by Stevenson, Hess, and Rheingold. New York: John Wiley & Sons, 1967.

Pearce, Joseph Chilton. *The Crack in the Cosmic Egg.* New York: Julian Press, 1971.

———. *Exploring the Crack in the Cosmic Egg.* New York: Julian Press, 1974.

Penfield, Wilder. *The Mystery of the Mind: A Critical Study of Consciousness and the Human Brain.* Princeton: Princeton University Press, 1975.

Peterson, James. "An Ignored Reality? Extrasensory Ability of Children." *Learning,* December 1975.

———. *Some Profiles of Non-ordinary Perception of Children.* Seminar Study for the Degree of Master of Arts. University of California, Berkeley, 1974.

Piaget, Jean. *Biology and Knowledge.* Chicago: University of Chicago Press, 1971.

———. *The Child's Conception of the World.* New York Humanities Press, 1951.

———. *Judgment and Reasoning in the Child.* Atlantic Highlands, N.J.: Humanities Press, 1952.

———. *The Origins of Intelligence in Children.* New York: International Universities Press, 1952.

———. *Play, Dreams and Imitation in Childhood.* New York: W. W. Norton & Company, 1962.

Piaget, J., and Inhelder, B. *The Early Growth of Logic in the Child.* Atlantic Highlands, N.J.: Humanities Press, 1964.

———. *The Psychology of the Child.* New York: Basic Books, 1969.

Polansky, Norman, et. al. *Profile of Neglect: A Survey of the State of Knowledge of Child Neglect.* Washington, D.C.: Department of Health, Education, and Welfare, Community Services Administration, 1975.

Prescott, James W. "Body Pleasure and the Origins of Violence." *The Futurist,* April 1975.

Pribram, Karl. *Language of the Brain.* Englewood Cliffs, N.J.: Prentice-Hall, 1971.

Rawls, John. *A Theory of Justice.* Cambridge, Mass.: Harvard University Press, 1971.

Rensberger, Boyce. "Earlier Evolution Suggested for Human Language and Intellectual Ability." *New York Times,* 25 September 1975.

Ribble, Margaret A. *The Rights of Infants.* New York: Columbia University Press, 1943.

Richards, M. P. M. "The Development of Psychological Communication in the First Year of Life." In *The Growth of Competence,* edited by Kevin Connolly and J. Bruner, pp. 119–132. New York: Academic Press, 1974.

Rimland, Bernard. *Infantile Autism.* New York: Appleton-Century-Crofts, 1964.

Robbins, Jeff. "Some Neuro-Physiological and Biochemical Aspects of Human Experience." Unpublished paper, San Francisco, May 1976.

Rochlin, Gregory. "The Dread of Abandonment: A Contribution to the Etiology of the Loss Complex and to Depression." In *The Psychoanalytic Study of the Child,* vol. 16, edited by Ruth Eisler. New York: International Universities Press, 1961.

———. "Fears of Death and Religious Beliefs." In *Griefs and Discontents.* Boston: Little, Brown and Company, 1975.

Rosenzweig, et al. "Brain Changes in Response to Experience." *Scientific American,* February 1972, pp. 22–29.

Ross, John. "The Resources of Binocular Perception in the Visual System." *Scientific American,* March 1976, pp. 80–86.

Samples, Robert E., *Toward a Synergy of Mind: Psychological Premises for Education before 1984.* Essentia, private printing. Evergreen State College, 1974.

Sannella, Lee, M.D. *Psychosis or Transcendence?* Berkeley, Calif.: private printing, 1975.

Schragg, P., and Divoky, D. *The Myth of the Hyperactive Child and Other Means of Child Control.* New York: Pantheon Books, 1975.

Selye, Hans. *The Stress of Life.* New York: McGraw-Hill Book Company, 1956.

Sperry, Roger. "Apparent Doubling of Consciousness in each Hemisphere." *American Psychologist* 23, no. 10 (October 1968).

Spitz, Renee. *The First Year of Life: A Psychoanalytic Study of Normal and Deviant*

Development of Object Relations. New York: International Universities Press, 1965.

Stace, Walter. *The Teachings of the Mystics.* New York: New American Library, 1960.

Steinberg, Saul. "The Brain as Supercomputer." *Brain-Mind Bulletin* no. 1.

Sullivan, Harry Stack. *The Interpersonal Theory of Psychiatry.* New York: W. W. Norton 1953.

Tart, Charles. *Altered States of Consciousness.* New York: John Wiley & Sons, 1969.

——. "Models for the Explanation of Extrasensory Perception." *International Journal of Neuropsychiatry* (1966).

——. "Physiological Correlates of Psi Cognition." *International Journal of Neuropsychiatry* 5, no. 4 (1962).

——. *States of Consciousness.* New York: E. P. Dutton, 1975.

Thrush, Ursulla. *Cosmic Education according to Montessori.* Syllabus. Sonoma, Calif.: Sonoma State College Extension Course, Sonma, Calif.

Tinbergen, Nikos. "Ethology and Stress Disease" *Science,* 5 July 1974, pp. 20–27.

Toulmin, Stephen. "Neuroscience and Human Understanding." In *The Neurosciences,* edited by G. C. Quarton. New York: Rockefeller University Press, 1967.

Vargui, James G. *A Model of Creative Behavior.* Redwood City, Calif.: Psychosynthesis Institute, 1973.

von Senden, M. *Space and Sight: The Perception of Space and Shape in the Congenitally Blind before and after Operation.* London: Methuen, 1960.

White, Burton L. *The First Three Years of Life.* Englewood Cliffs, N.J.: Prentice-Hall, 1975.

——. *Human Infants: Experience and Psychological Development.* Englewood Cliffs, N.J.: Prentice-Hall, 1971.

Wickes, Frances. *The Inner World of Childhood.* New York: Appleton-Century-Crofts 1968.

Wiener, Joan, and Glick, Joyce. *Adventures in Pregnancy: Birth and Being a Mother.* New York: Collier Books, 1974.

Windle, W. F. "Brain Damage by Asphyxia." *Scientific American,* October 1969, pp. 76–84.

Yogananda, Paramahansa. *Autobiography of a Yogi.* Los Angeles: Self-Realization Fellowship, 1946.

Zaslow, R. W. *The Psychology of the Z-Process: Attachment and Activation.* Private printing. San Jose State University, 1975.

——. *Resistance to Human Attachment and Growth: Autism to Retardation.* Los Gatos, Calif.: Nova Press, 1970.

Zaslow, R. W., and Breger, L. "A Theory and Treatment of Autism." In *Clinical-Cognitive Psychology: Models and Integration,* edited by L. Breger. Englewood Cliffs, N.J.: Prentice-Hall, 1969.

Zipf, George Kingsley. *Human Behavior and the Principle of Least Resistance: An Introduction to Human Ecology.* Reading, Mass.: Addison-Wesley Publishing Co., 1949.

——. *The Psycho Biology of Language: An Introduction to Dynamic Philology.* Cambridge, Mass.: M.I.T. Press, 1965.

Subject Bibliography

Autism, Psychosis, and General Damage
Becker, *The Revolution in Psychiatry;* Gardner, "Deprivation Dwarfism"; Harlow and Harlow, "Social Deprivation in Monkeys"; Kaufman and Rosenbloom, "Depression in Infant Monkeys"; Massie, "The Early Natural History of Childhood Psychosis"; Massie, "Patterns of Mother-Infant Behavior and Subsequent Childhood Psychosis"; Prescott, "Body Pleasure and the Origins of Violence"; Robbins, "Some Neuro-Physiological and Biochemical Aspects of Human Experience"; Rochlin, "The Dread of Abandonment"; Sannella, *Psychosis or Transcendence?;* Schragg and Divoky, *The Myth of the Hyperactive Child and Other Means of Child Control;* Tinbergen, "Ethology and Stress Disease"; Windle, "Brain Damage by Asphyxia"; Zaslow, *The Psychology of the Z-Process;* Zaslow, *Resistance to Human Attachment and Growth;* Zaslow and Breger, "A Theory and Treatment of Autism."

Bonding (Attachment)
Ainsworth, "Deprivation of Maternal Care"; Ainsworth, *Infancy in Uganda,* Ainsworth, "Patterns of Attachment Behavior Shown by the Infant in Interaction with His Mother"; Bowlby, "The Child's Tie to His Mother"; Bowlby, "Maternal Care and Mental Health"; Bowlby, "Separation Anxiety"; Gardner, "Deprivation Dwarfism"; Geber, "The Psycho-Motor Development of African Children in the First Year and the Influence of Maternal Behavior"; Harlow, "Love in Infant Monkeys"; Jones, *Ethological Studies of Child Behavior;* Klaus, "Human Maternal Behavior at the First Contact with Her Young"; Klaus, "Maternal Attachment."

Brain, Physiology, and Learning Mechanism

Aaron, "The World of the Brain"; Bengeldorf, "Neural Mechanisms of Learning and Memory"; Ehrenwald, "Brain Model for Processing Psychic Events"; Epstein, "Phrenoblysis: Special Brain and Mind Growth Periods"; Ferguson, *The Brain Revolution;* Gregory, *Eye and Brain;* John, "How the Brain Works —A New Theory"; Luria, *The Role of Speech in Normal and Abnormal Behavior;* Ornstein, *The Psychology of Consciousness;* Penfield, *The Mystery of the Mind;* Piaget, *Biology and Knowledge;* Pribram, *Language of the Brain;* Rensberger, "Earlier Evolution Suggested for Human Language and Intellectual Ability"; Robbins, "Some Neuro-Physiological and Biochemical Aspects of Human Experience"; Rosenzweig, "Brain Changes in Response to Experience"; Ross, "The Resources of Binocular Perception in the Visual System"; Steinberg, "The Brain as Supercomputer"; Tart, *States of Consciousness;* Vargui, *A Model of Creative Behavior;* von Senden, *Space and Sight.*

Causality (Scientists on the Relation between Mind, Reality, and Matter)

Bohm, *Causality and Chance in Modern Physics;* Bohm, "Reality and Knowledge Considered as Process"; Burgers, "Causality and Anticipation"; Chomsky, "Recent Contributions to the Theory of Innate Ideas"; Globus, "Unexpected Symmetries in the 'World Knot' "; Josephson, "Possible Connections between Psychic Phenomena and Quantum Mechanics"; Toulmin, "Neuroscience and Human Understanding."

Child Intelligence

Almy, *Young Children's Thinking;* Beadle, *A Child's Mind;* Beck, *How to Raise a Brighter Child* (typical mid-1950s "how to make your offspring the fastest gun on the block"—that is, street smart in the sematic world); Bruner, *Beyond the Information Given;* Bruner, "Processes of Growth in Infancy"; Bruner, Goodnow, and Austin, *A Study of Thinking;* Burke, "Two Orders of Learning"; Flavell, *The Developmental Psychology of Jean Piaget;* Greenfield, "Curriculum for the Day Care Center at Boston's Bromley-Heath"; Harwood, *The Way of a Child;* Jones, *Ethological Studies of Child Behavior;* Wickes, *The Inner World of Childhood.*

Cross-Cultural

Ainsworth, *Infancy in Uganda;* Bateson, *Steps to an Ecology of Mind;* Belo, *Trance in Bali;* Carpenter, *Eskimo Realities;* Carpenter, *Oh, What a Blow That Phantom Gave Me!;* Jones, *Ethological Studies of Child Behavior.*

Death, Abandonment, and Anxiety

Anthony, *The Child's Discovery of Death;* Bowlby, "Process of Mourning"; Brody and Axelrod, *Anxiety and Ego Formation in Infancy;* Kaufman and Rosenbloom, "Depression in Infant Monkeys"; Maurer, "Maturation of Concepts of Death"; Rochlin, "The Dread of Abandonment"; Rochlin, "Fears of Death and Religious Beliefs."

Dreams

Faraday, *The Dream Game;* Fisher, "A Psychophysiological Study of Nightmares and Night Terrors"; Foulkes, "Longitudinal Studies of Dreams in Children"; Milton Stewart in Tart, *Altered States of Consciousness.*

General

Carpenter, *Eskimo Realities;* Chomsky, "Recent Contributions to the Theory of Innate Ideas"; Kellog, *Analyzing Children's Art;* Kessen, *Childhood in*

China; Koestler, *The Act of Creation;* Polansky, *Profile of Neglect;* Rawls, *A Theory of Justice;* Selye, *The Stress of Life;* Tinbergen, "Ethology and Stress Disease"; Vargui, *A Model of Creative Behavior;* Yogananda, *Autobiography of a Yogi,* Zipf, *Human Behavior and the Principle of Least Resistance;* Zipf, *The Psycho Biology of Language.*

Infant Intelligence

Ainsworth; *Infancy in Uganda;* Almy, *Young Children's Thinking;* Beadle, *A Child's Mind;* Geber, "The Psycho-Motor Development of African Children in the First Year and the Influence of Maternal Behavior"; Gray, "Imprinting in Infants"; Hess and Shipman, "Early Experiences and the Socialization of the Cognitive Modes in Children"; Jones, *Ethological Studies of Child Behavior;* Lake, "New Babies Are Smarter Than You Think"; LeBoyer, *Birth without Violence;* Papousek, "Experimental Studies of Appetitional Behavior in Human Newborns and Infants"; Ribble, *The Rights of Infants;* Richards, "The Development of Psychological Communication in the First Year of Life"; Spitz, *The First Year of Life;* White, *Human Infants.*

Language

Bernard and Sontag, "Fetal Reactions to Sound"; Cassierer, *Language and Myth;* Condon and Sander, "Neonate Movement Is Synchronized with Adult Speech"; Fodor, "Speech Discrimination in Infants"; Furth, *Deafness and Learning;* Furth, *Thinking without Language;* Rensberger, "Earlier Evolution Suggested for Human Language and Intellectual Ability"; Zipf, *The Psycho Biology of Language.*

Male-Female

Gilder, *Naked Nomads* (selections); MacKellar, *Rape: The Bait and the Trap;* Montagu, *The Natural Superiority of Women.*

Nonordinary Phenomena

Belo, *Trance in Bali;* Ehrenwald, "Brain Model for Processing Psychic Events"; Feinberg, "Firewalking in Ceylon"; Manning, *The Link;* Monroe, *Journeys Out of the Body;* Nakaoka, "Parapsychological Argument in Japan"; Ostrander and Schroder, *Psychic Discoveries behind the Iron Curtain;* Panati, *Geller Papers;* Pearce, *The Crack in the Cosmic Egg;* Peterson, "An Ignored Reality?"; Peterson, *Some Profiles of Non-ordinary Perception of Children;* Tart, *Altered States of Consciousness;* Tart, "Models for the Explanation of Extrasensory Perception"; Tart, "Physiological Correlates of Psi Cognition"; Tart, *States of Consciousness.*

Parent-Child

Cooper, *The Death of the Family* (to deny the validity of the nuclear parental bond is to err grievously); Ginott, *Between Parent and Child;* Ginott, *Between Parent and Teenager* (decent, solid man); Gordon, *P.E.T.* (typical prescriptions trying to cover the infinitely variable facets of the monstrous misunderstanding); Lowry, "Environmental Influences on Measures of Intelligence"; Lowry, "First-Borns with Siblings vs. First-Borns without Siblings"; White, *The First Three Years of Life* (had White not assumed the institutionalized child the norm and so underestimated the importance of the early bonding period, his work would have been stronger; also he tries to prescribe specific actions).

Piaget

His own works: *Biology and Knowledge; The Child's Conception of the World; Judgment and Reasoning in the Child; The Origins of Intelligence in Children; Play, Dreams and Imitation in Childhood;* with Imhelder: *The Early Growth of Logic in the Child; The Psychology of the Child;* studies of Piaget's theory (much easier to approach): Almy, *Young Children's Thinking;* Flavell, *The Developmental Psychology of Jean Piaget;* Furth, *Piaget and Knowledge;* Furth, *Piaget for Teachers.*

Play

Csikszentmihalyi, "Play and Intrinsic Rewards" (one of the most impressive papers I received and a key synthesis to the magical child); Curtis, "Aikido" (speaks of the same flow ecstacy found in play); Piaget, *Play, Dreams and Imitation in Childhood.*

Prenatal and Delivery

Ainsworth, "Deprivation of Maternal Care"; Ainsworth, *Infancy in Uganda;* Ainsworth, "Patterns of Attachment Behavior Shown by the Infant in Interaction with His Mother"; Arms, *Immaculate Deception;* Bernard and Sontag, "Fetal Reactions to Sound"; Bowlby, "The Child's Tie to His Mother"; Bowlby, "Maternal Care and Mental Health"; Cheek, "Maladjustments May Be Results of Birth Events"; Condon and Sander "Neonate Movement Is Synchronized with Adult Speech"; Connolly and Bruner, *The Growth of Competence;* Farnsworth, "Reach Out for the Hours After Birth"; Geber, "The Psycho-Motor Development of African Children in the First Year and the Influence of Maternal Behavior"; Gray, "Imprinting in Infants"; Jones, *Ethological Studies of Child Behavior;* Klaus, "Human Maternal Behavior at the First Contact with Her Young"; Klaus, "Maternal Attachment"; Lake, "New Babies Are Smarter Than You Think"; LeBoyer, *Birth without Violence;* Levine, "Stimulation in Infancy"; Montagu, *Life before Birth;* Montagu, *Prenatal Influences;* Montagu, *Touching;* Prescott, "Body Pleasure and the Origins of Violence"; Ribble, *The Rights of Infants;* Richards, "The Development of Psychological Communications in the First Year of Life"; Wiener and Glick, *Adventures in Pregnancy.*

Primate Correlations

Harlow, "Love in Infant Monkeys"; Harlow and Harlow, "Social Deprivation in Monkeys"; Kaufman and Rosenbloom, "Depression in Infant Monkeys"; Mitchell, "What Monkeys Can Tell Us about Human Violence."

Psychology, Psychiatry

Becker, *The Denial of Death;* Becker, *The Revolution in Psychiatry;* Sannella, *Psychosis or Transcendence?* Sullivan, *The Interpersonal Theory of Psychiatry;* Wickes, *The Inner World of Childhood;* Zaslow, *The Psychology of the Z-Process.*

Right-Left Brain Hemispheres

Bruner, *On Knowing;* Burke, "Two Orders of Learning"; Hilgard, "Hypnosis Is No Mirage"; Hilgard, *Hypnotic Susceptibility;* Hilgard, "Two Separate Cognitive Systems;" Ornstein, *The Nature of Human Consciousness;* Ornstein, *The Psychology of Consciousness;* Samples, *Toward a Synergy of Mind;* Sperry, "Apparent Doubling of Consciousness in Each Hemisphere"; Tart, *States of Consciousness.*

School

Bruner, *Beyond the Information Given;* Bruner, *The Relevance of Education;* Holt, *Instead of Education* (I wish Holt had said "schooling" rather than "education." We need, but do not have, education. His critique of schooling is marvelous.); Thrush, *Cosmic Education according to Montessori.*

Skin Stimulus and the Newborn

Levine, "Stimulation and Infancy"; Massie, "The Early Natural History of Childhood Psychosis"; Massie, "Patterns of Mother-Infant Behavior and Subsequent Childhood Psychosis"; Montagu, *Touching;* Prescott, "Body Pleasure and the Origins of Violence."

Vision

Bowlby, "The Child's Tie to His Mother"; Fantz, "The Origin of Form Perception"; Fantz, "Pattern Vision in Young Infants"; Gregory, *Eye and Brain;* Ross; The Resources of Binocular Perception in the Visual System"; von Senden, *Space and Sight.*

Index